UN-ADDICTION

UN-ADDICTION

6 MIND-CHANGING CONVERSATIONS THAT COULD SAVE A LIFE

NZINGA HARRISON, MD
WITH LYNYA FLOYD

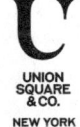

UNION SQUARE & CO.
NEW YORK

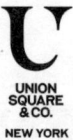

UNION SQUARE & CO.
NEW YORK

UNION SQUARE & CO. and the distinctive Union Square & Co. logo
are trademarks of Sterling Publishing Co., Inc.

Union Square & Co., LLC, is a subsidiary of Sterling Publishing Co., Inc.

Text and author photo © 2024 Nzinga Harrison

All rights reserved. No part of this publication may be reproduced, stored
in a retrieval system, or transmitted in any form or by any means
(including electronic, mechanical, photocopying, recording, or otherwise)
without prior written permission from the publisher.

The information in this book is intended for informational or educational purposes
only. This book is not intended or implied to be a substitute for professional medical
advice, diagnosis, or treatment. All content, including text, graphics, images, and
information contained herein is for general information purposes only and is offered
with no guarantees. The author and publisher disclaim all liability in connection
with the use of this book and the material it contains.

The author and editor have made every effort to reproduce the substance of the
conversations relied on in this book but some have been edited and condensed for
clarity and space. Names and identifying details have been changed at the individuals'
request and/or to preserve the author's obligation to uphold patient confidentiality.

ISBN 978-1-4549-5555-9

First published in the United Kingdom in 2024 by Union Square & Co., LLC.

A catalogue record of this book is available from the British Library.

For information about custom editions, special sales, and premium purchases,
please contact specialsales@unionsquareandco.com.

Printed in the United Kingdom

2 4 6 8 10 9 7 5 3 1

unionsquareandco.com

Cover design by Elizabeth Milhaltse Lindy
Interior design by Kevin Ullrich

Image credits appear on page 264

For every person who has struggled to find compassion, connection, and hope in the face of addiction.

CONTENTS

Preface viii

Introduction 1

PART I: The Addiction Risks We Inherit 16

Chapter One: Why Some Monkeys Can't Lay Off the Mojitos 19
> *The surprising ways DNA impacts the biological risk of substance use*

Chapter Two: The Accidental Discovery of an Addiction Predictor............. 57
> *Tell me about your childhood, and I'll tell you about your addiction risk*

Chapter Three: A Garden of Eden for Rats................................... 94
> *Why environment matters when it comes to substance use*

PART II: The Addiction Risks We Acquire 126

Chapter Four: Is Finding a Man the Solution for Jan?...................... 129
> *Three prescription pills and one big problem*

Chapter Five: How Weathering Any Storm Can Wither Your Health........... 164
> *Adversity increases your chances of chronic illness*

Chapter Six: Scrolling Toward Addiction 197
> *From social media to national holidays–the cultures and environments that encourage risky substance use*

Conclusion 232
Recommended Resources... 236
Appendix 238
Notes 241
Image Credits 264
Acknowledgments 265
Index 267
About the Author.. 272

PREFACE

I'm about to tell you some stories that will surprise you. Eye-opening stories you'll find hard to believe that are rooted in research and supported by studies but rarely told. Stories about alcoholic monkeys that get into the equivalent of bar fights on the beaches of St. Kitts and a blood-free test you've never heard of that predicts the likelihood of you struggling with addiction.

I'm about to tell you some stories that will upset you at first. Heart-wrenching stories of my patients whose substance use resulted in terrible outcomes. Stories about broken relationships that were mended, and lives set off course that got back on track with compassionate care.

I'm about to tell you some stories that will empower you. Inspiring stories that will give you the exact tools you need to support loved ones who struggle with substance use. Stories that will help you all move forward instead of feeling stuck in the cycle of addiction.

But first, I'm going to tell you a story about parking my car.

A few years back, I was running late for an expensive business dinner at an expensive restaurant at an expensive hotel in downtown Atlanta. As I handed over my keys, I let my glance linger a little as the valet exclaimed, "Dr. Harrison?!"

PREFACE

At that moment, it hit me why he looked so familiar. I remembered him as one of my patients from a clinic where I had served as the director and treating psychiatrist for hundreds of people seeking recovery from drugs and alcohol. I was looking into the eyes of a success story.

A smile fell over my face because he was, as I like to call it, "thriving." When someone is struggling with substance use, they look to me like a plant that is withering because it hasn't gotten enough water or sunlight. But when I see people in recovery, I witness those leaves coming back to lush greenery and beginning to not just survive—but thrive. That was this man. I noticed how happy he looked. His skin was glowing and there was some pep in his step as he confidently moved forward to give me a big hug.

"I've been clean for the last five years!" he proudly said.

I winced inwardly at the use of the word "clean," fully aware of the connotation that people with active addiction are inherently "dirty," but I let it roll off and hugged him back tightly.

Suddenly, not caring that I was running late, I spent several minutes catching up with him and reveling in the success and life meaning he'd found, despite all odds being stacked against him. He had been able to maintain complete abstinence for several years and was proud to be working two jobs—one as a valet, and the other as a personal trainer. He was going to Narcotics Anonymous meetings. His relationships were coming back to him. In truth, his whole life was coming back to him.

As a Black man born into poverty and snatched up by the criminal justice system at an early age, who had struggled with addiction for

PREFACE

most of his young life, I knew he had been dealt a bad hand and that standing in front of me was a wonder to behold. I wasn't going to miss the opportunity to tell him as much. He was a success story, but he wasn't an anomaly. A full 75 percent of Americans with substance use disorders are in recovery or recovered—especially if they get good treatment. That's an incredible fact that nobody would ever guess.

"I'll never forget how you made us all feel like you really cared," he said.

"Because I really did!" I replied. "I care about each and every one of you."

It was not lost on me how sad an indictment his statement was about the way doctors, family, friends, and lovers can treat those with addiction. It's easy to make someone with addiction feel as if you don't care about them—even when you care so much it hurts. The ways we've been taught to show we care—tough love, confrontational interventions, letting a person who is using hit rock bottom—are actually hurtful. The truth is that many people care about those with addiction, but most of them don't know how to show it.

I darted off to my meeting teary-eyed. I was filled with a mixture of hope for this man's individual fortitude and anger at the racist, oppressive, socially unjust America that would systematically threaten his sobriety each day going forward. I was also aware that there would be threats to his sobriety from within—right down to the cellular level. Biologically, his DNA had not only increased his risk of addiction but was also working against him now that even the synapses in his brain had grown accustomed to controlled substances. Psychologically, a childhood of poverty and mistreatment from his mother's revolving

PREFACE

door of boyfriends coded anxiety, fear, and hypervigilance into his very being. He would likely always be fighting an inner voice that critically asked him, "What makes you think you deserve a good life? What makes you think you can get ahead?" Environmentally, he was living in a culture where everything from our fireworks-laden holidays to our chart-topping popular songs celebrate drinking and using drugs.

Still, he found hope. He persisted. He joined the 75 percent. And he's the success story I'm telling you now so that you're aware of what is possible, probable, and, shockingly, left unspoken.

We're silent about addiction in so many ways. We're not only quiet about the success stories, but we also feel like we need to keep it a secret when someone we love is in the midst of a struggle. So, let's talk about some of the numbers that are hard to hear.

The Impact of Addiction

In the United States, 46 percent of adults have a family member or close friend who is or has been addicted to drugs. Or should we say 46 percent of us are willing to admit it in a poll? Add alcohol to the equation and that number undoubtedly skyrockets. That means addiction touches the lives of more than one hundred million Americans every single year.

We all know what that looks like. It's our neighbor who quietly recycles their bottles and cans when no one is around to judge. A brother who disappears into the bathroom a little too often at Thanksgiving. A teenager who buys pain pills from their friend after school. Ourselves, craving Cab Sauvignon or edibles every Friday by 5:01 p.m.

PREFACE

And yet, *somehow*, we think that 46 percent is everybody else. We've let addiction become an open secret in America. But it is way past time we stop talking about it in hushed tones and start addressing it with full-voiced, wholehearted, and deeply compassionate solutions.

For years, I've wanted to write a book for each of these people I've just described and the people whose lives they've touched. A book for any person who ever wondered why their partner can't just stop drinking, why their teenager would risk jail for another hit, why their favorite celebrity just can't seem to pull it together—or why they can't seem to pull it together themselves. For everyone who reads it, I hope this book will provide not only insight, but also inspiration and life-changing ideas on how relationships and lives can be saved.

The answer to this addiction crisis, in so many ways, is to deepen your understanding of substance use as a chronic illness and not a moral failing. I can say without a doubt that addiction is one of the most misunderstood chronic medical conditions of our lifetime. That's why I titled this book *Un-Addiction*. You're about to unlearn everything that you think you know about addiction. For example, roughly 30 percent of Americans believe recovery from drug addiction is impossible. They reject the idea that treatment can enable someone to get well and go on to live a productive life. Having only read this far, you already know that's not true. You know about the 75 percent success rate. You know that cutting ties, packing up bags, and giving up hope is not necessary or helpful. So, we're making progress already. But there's more I want to share.

What if I told you that the one-year relapse rates for high blood pressure and asthma were the same as or higher than the relapse rates

PREFACE

for addiction? And that means there's a greater chance of your blood pressure or breathing being out of control after a treatment intervention than your drug use being out of control after rehab or another treatment intervention? Would you say, "Stop treating blood pressure and asthma because those people don't want to get better, and treatment doesn't work anyway"? Never. And yet that is what we are saying about addiction. We are actively undermining the most important element of recovery: hope. By doing so, we are all but ensuring that people will continue to die from addiction—hopeless and untreated.

The good news is that we don't have to stay on this hopeless path. We don't have to keep watching our neighbors, siblings, partners, kids, colleagues, and friends suffer and die. We can, and must, start giving hope back. We can unlearn what we erroneously yet deeply believe about addiction. We can undo the stigma surrounding addiction and treatment. We can undertake hard but rewarding conversations that can affect lasting change on ourselves and in our loved ones. I'm looking forward to giving you the tools to do this. As a board-certified doctor in both adult general psychiatry and addiction medicine, I've spent my career treating individuals with substance use disorders and other mental health conditions from trauma, depression, and anxiety to bipolar disorder and schizophrenia. In that time, I've not only come to understand the complex factors that put us all at risk for addiction, but I've also uncovered the combination of interventions most likely to help a person recover from it. I'm going to share the factors that put us at risk here. In turn, I hope you'll do the work and share it with others because I've seen the power that it has to actually save lives that might otherwise be lost.

PREFACE

Why I Do What I Do

I became interested in addiction medicine for a simple reason: Nobody wanted to spend time with "drug addicts" when I was in medical school. They're among the most marginalized and mistreated groups by the medical system. If psychiatry and mental health are the redheaded stepchildren of medicine, then addiction is the redheaded stepchild of the redheaded stepchild. Nobody wanted to get involved with these human beings going through a struggle. But I did. I could see my family in so many of the patients I worked with.

Now that I'm a psychiatrist, I can see my family tree made me destined to be an addiction specialist. I think about my mean-as-hell paternal grandmother sending me to the grocery store as a child to pick up gold cans that said "BEER." I think of my aunt and favorite uncle, whose cocaine addictions were severe. My aunt's led to her abandoning my cousins. My uncle struggled so much that at holiday dinners, all the women would lock up their purses in my grandmother's bedroom so he couldn't comb through them for drug money. My maternal grandmother showed compassion but also set healthy boundaries that kept the family safe. "You can always come home," she told my uncle. "But you can't live here." At the time of this book, my aunt has been in recovery for twenty-two years and my uncle is working hard and getting healthier day by day.

Sadly, families can struggle just as much as the medical system to provide the support people with active addiction need. I saw this as a fourth-year medical student on the liver transplant psychiatry team. We made recommendations about which terminally ill patients should

PREFACE

be added to the wait list for a new liver. One of the health requirements for being placed on the list is that you be someone who never used alcohol or other drugs or someone in remission for at least three years. The remission criterion made sense to me because alcohol and other drugs can be very damaging to the liver. But I quickly came to notice that patients with other diseases that also could be very damaging to the liver were not held to the same standards. The dirty little secret is that even if you were in recovery for years, you still might not get on the list.

There was no equity. Addiction wasn't being treated like other diseases. It was on this rotation that I started to draw the conclusion that the lives of people who use alcohol and drugs don't matter to the healthcare system.

As part of the transplant psychiatry team, I'd comb through thick case files at the hospital looking for all the reasons I could find to fight hard to get someone who had suffered from alcohol use disorder on the list. It took an extraordinary amount of work, education, and advocacy to make the review board know: "This isn't a bad person making bad choices." We were making life-and-death arguments for people and that weighed heavily on me.

The response from the review board was often the same. "Will they start drinking again? Can we take that chance?" the board would ask. They'd essentially turn addiction into a scarlet letter you'd have to wear for the rest of your life. No fresh start. No place—even at the back of the line.

It was on that rotation I knew I could make a real impact. I realized the system is not only killing people with substance use disorders, but

PREFACE

also poor people, people of color, all people. It's killing people that life has already dealt a very terrible hand. The very people that we should be helping the most. And it doesn't care.

All my professional life, I've been fighting for people struggling with substance use from inside the health system. With this book, I hope to help them win outside of the system as well. I wrote this book because I want anyone who struggles with substance use to become a better advocate for themselves and for their loved ones who may be struggling. I hope to radically change the way that you look at, talk about, and react to addiction and substance use. I'm going to explain how to go from someone who doesn't know how to show you care for someone with addiction to becoming someone who does. That way, maybe, when someone thanks you for caring and supporting them in recovery one day, you won't be saddened a little, like I was when I spoke to the valet. Together we're going to create the change that we want to see in the world of substance use. And we're going to do it one family at a time.

INTRODUCTION

Before I can start to change the way you think about addiction, we first have to talk about the definition of addiction. When I speak to high school students about what addiction is, I ask them to share their definitions with me on an electronic chalkboard. It never ceases to amaze me how many of them have been touched by addiction through their family members, how many of them have already thought about what it means, and how many of them express some heartbreaking, personal connection to what they've written on the board. When I talk about addiction, I refer to the official definition from the American Society of Addiction Medicine, a professional medical society for more than 7,000 physicians, clinicians, and associated professionals in the field of addiction medicine. Their words, my bolding:

> Addiction is a **treatable**, chronic **medical disease** involving complex interactions among brain circuits, genetics, the environment, and an individual's life experiences. People with addiction use substances or engage in behaviors that become **compulsive** and often continue despite **harmful consequences**.

INTRODUCTION

Let's break this down. First, addiction is treatable. As I mentioned earlier, 75 percent of Americans with substance use disorders are in recovery. Next, it's a chronic medical disease—it's not a choice or a moral failure. There is something occurring in the brains of people with addiction that differs from those without. Finally, it's compulsive and has harmful consequences. Like cleaning, re-cleaning, and re-cleaning a countertop when you have an obsessive-compulsive disorder, addiction, too, is hard to control.

A simpler way of talking about addiction risk is by looking at biological, psychological, and environmental influences. Every state of illness or wellness has biological, psychological, and environmental inputs. Every single one—not just addiction. And for each of those inputs, there are inherited factors that you're born with or experience as a child and acquired factors you are exposed to when you're older (see the graphic on the following page). Over the course of this book, I will walk you through all six of these factors that can contribute to your risk of any illness, but particularly to substance use disorders. If we're trying to make the biggest, most positive impact on our health and empower ourselves to achieve wellness goals, we have to take a look at each of these six inputs.

As you make your way through each chapter, I have two asks: Take your time and keep an open mind. You're going to be presented with research, statistics, and true stories that will likely be contrary to everything you ever thought or were told about addiction. That's because from "Just Say No" campaigns to depictions of addiction on wildly popular TV shows, most of what you've been taught about addiction, what you've been shown about people who use drugs, and what you've

INTRODUCTION

Addiction Risk Factors

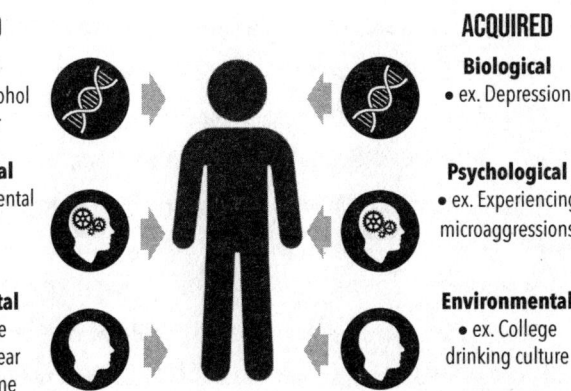

been told about prescription and illicit drugs, is wrong. But we're about to make things right.

By understanding the impact of your biological, psychological, and environmental inputs, you can harness that knowledge to maximize the factors that work *for* you and minimize those that are working *against* you using homework that I'll give you at the end of each chapter. The homework will create what I call your Magic Formula™ for health, a personalized plan to intervene in each of those areas—reinforcing the input if it's positive and seeking to make a change if it's not. No two Magic Formulas™ are the same, because no two people have the exact same combination of biological, psychological, and environmental inherited and acquired factors. As one of my math-nerd friends would say: it's statistically improbable!

Each of those influences is like a strand in an intricately crafted web. And that internal web of ours is connected to an infinite number of

INTRODUCTION

external webs: the webs of the other people we live with, work with, play with, and travel with. The webs of the experiences we have in life and those of the environments we encounter. So, you're never really just looking at one input. You're looking at how all of the connections link together to form the big picture. Now that I've explained the strands of the web separately, let's look at an example of how they surprisingly connect to each other and sometimes work together to undermine your health outcomes. Let's start with a chronic health condition like asthma.

Imagine you have a son in the first grade who is running around and giggling at the playground with his friends—but then begins slowing down and looking more serious as he struggles to catch his breath. Worried, you take your child to the doctor to find out that he's one of the roughly six million children in the United States who have asthma, a chronic lung disease that inflames the airways of the lungs, making it harder to bring air in and out of the body.

"Why my kid? How did this happen?" you ask your doctor, as she shares a laundry list of things that you couldn't control: Your child being male, Black, and maybe your husband having childhood asthma that he forgot to tell you about. Family history, gender, and race are all *inherited biological factors* that can increase the risk of developing childhood asthma. But so do other things that we are not born with. Maybe you tried to move to a "better" neighborhood when your kid was born—a building that wasn't constructed with cheap, questionable materials or an apartment that didn't have paper-thin walls that allowed your neighbor's cigarette smoke to creep in. Hearing that growing up in a low-income area and being exposed to tobacco smoke

INTRODUCTION

are *inherited environmental risk factors* could cause you to put the blame on yourself because your kid will always have to travel with an inhaler.

You may then try to explain in simple terms to your child why they have very scary moments of not being able to catch their breath. Maybe your son's anxiety kicks in every time he has recess at school because he anticipates his lungs closing up on the next round of tag or kickball. Maybe he's nervous on that school trip to the botanical gardens because he knows that flowers and allergens could trigger an asthma attack. That increased stress then triggers symptoms so he starts using his rescue inhaler a little more often, which can actually lead to more frequent and worse asthma symptoms. That's *acquired psychological* (fear) and *acquired biological* (the inhaler) factors interacting and putting him at risk for worsening asthma.

Then perhaps when you take him to the doctor, you both experience discrimination and he's not able to get the care he deserves. Or you worry about the family dynamics that your son fits into (or doesn't) if he's viewed as weaker than his siblings or his cousins because his asthma prevents him from excelling at sports. That's *acquired environmental risk*.

All of this is a lot for this mom to deal with. And I imagine you naturally felt a lot of compassion and understanding for her and her son as you read their story.

That's the same compassion and understanding that I'm hoping this book will bring you as you learn about the factors that can lead to a substance use disorder. Let's say instead of a kid with asthma, you're dropping your teenage daughter off at a friend's house for a sleepover.

INTRODUCTION

Knowing that you had bouts of binge drinking all throughout your twenties, you worry about whether your child will also develop an alcohol use disorder. After all, research shows that up to 60 percent of the risk of developing a substance use disorder is inherited, so her family tree—with you being the nearest branch—means a lot.

But you haven't spoken with your daughter about your past. You think that she's seen enough of the violent fights between you and your ex, who has since left, to know that she shouldn't drink. Now we're tapping into *inherited psychological risk*. As you drive away from her friend's house, your heart sinks a bit as you become acutely aware of the state of your neighborhood, which has a liquor store on every third corner and is at least a twenty-minute drive to a safe park. What, you imagine, are your daughter and her friend going to do for fun all afternoon at that house? That's *inherited environmental risk*.

Beyond the inherited factors that can put your daughter at risk are the acquired ones. Maybe she heads off to college, but isn't accustomed to the work and pressure that come with it. Or perhaps there aren't many other Latinx students like her in her class and the microaggressions from her classmates are getting to her. She's starting to feel depressed and the only thing that seems to help is partying with people she hopes to befriend. She goes to keggers where there is plenty of heavy drinking that she eventually can't control. Her *acquired biology* (depression), *psychology* (discrimination), and *environment* (new school) have all dramatically increased her risk. Now you're picking her up mid-semester and signing her up for rehab.

If you've arrived at an equal level of compassion for the kid with asthma and the teen with an alcohol use disorder, I'm thankful.

INTRODUCTION

Compassion is the central theme of this book. I feel strongly that being able to understand what people are navigating and compassionately supporting them in doing so without judgment is the best chance we have to significantly reduce substance-related deaths and improve recovery rates. When you're sick—whether you have the flu or cocaine use disorder—you can't get better if people are being cruel to you. Telling someone to snap out of it or shaming them for their illness hurts far more than you probably realize. When you're not well, you need support above and beyond.

Outside of the six biological, psychological, and environmental inputs I'll be sharing, another way I'm going to help you think about addiction differently is by talking differently about it. Any subject you're learning about has a specific language tied to it. And addiction is no different. We're going to change the words that we use to discuss addiction—no longer, for example, referring to people in recovery as "clean" because the opposite of that would be "dirty." You wouldn't call someone struggling with asthma or diabetes or hypertension dirty until they got their condition under control. Or the way we now frequently use people-first language in healthcare, referring to someone as a person first and then naming their ailment second. We no longer talk about autistics, diabetics, or the blind. We now talk about people with autism, people with diabetes, and people who are blind.

The importance of language was never more apparent to me than one afternoon when I was staring intently at my work computer getting into the weeds of a study or some spreadsheet when a phone call broke my concentration. It was the mother of a former patient who had recently entered remission from cocaine addiction.

INTRODUCTION

"I know if my daughter gets a job while she's in recovery, she'll be a good person again," her mother pleaded to me. "Before she started using, she was brilliant, clever, and kind. She hasn't been using for two months now."

Here was this loving, super supportive mother willing to do whatever she could to help her child succeed. And yet, she was talking about her child in the past tense. The daughter *was* brilliant. She *was* a good person. It was as if her daughter had died, though she was still alive and beginning to thrive. This mother was confusing the symptoms of her daughter's illness with the permanent personal qualities that her daughter would have for a lifetime.

I was highly aware that she was pleading her daughter's case. She felt like she had to prove to me that her child was a good person—despite her addiction. But she shouldn't have to pull out all the stops for anyone—and especially not for me. I am the last person that needed to be convinced. I know from science, from experience, and from my heart that just because someone has an addiction doesn't mean they will forever make bad decisions, can't be trusted, or aren't a good person. But that is what most people think. The longer a person is in recovery, the easier it is for people to believe that someone has changed. It's not that the person has changed. It's that the symptoms of their illness are in remission. It's the same with cancer: the longer it's gone, the easier it is to believe that it won't come back.

Each time we use words or phrases that degrade or demean people with active addiction, we only make their recovery and sustained sobriety that much harder. We add to the deadly weight of stigma and detract from the understanding of addiction as a biological

INTRODUCTION

disease—not a desired choice. Words have psychological power. The words we use to describe addiction and those with addiction can either hurt or help those around us. Never has talking the talk been more important. If you're ready to be part of the solution, start working the following words and phrases into your vocabulary.

What You Used to Say:
"They abuse substances."

What You'll Say Going Forward:
"They engage in harmful substance use" or "They have a substance use disorder."

Abuse is a crime. Substance use disorder is an illness. Harmful substance use is an early warning sign of addiction. We're not talking about people committing crimes. We are talking about people suffering from an illness. When we use the term "abuse," we create stigma for those most in need of support and compassion instead.

Now let's address the other elephant in the room: there's an inherent bias in using the term "substance abuse" because people have ideas about acceptable and unacceptable drugs. I triple dare you to think of a time when someone used the words "substance abuse" while talking about someone on their fifth cosmo at dinner or their second cigarette of the morning, for example. After all, a mysterious woman in a dimly lit club drinking whiskey as a man leans over to light her cigarette is the quintessential, cool Hollywood scene, right? But heroin, methamphetamine, and inhalants? That's the "substance abuse" people easily refer

INTRODUCTION

to. Those are an entirely different type of quintessential movie scene that doesn't end with the steamy sex scene or the successful bank heist. That ending is usually pretty tragic.

For the record, medical professionals aren't immune to this kind of bias either. As recently as ten years ago, as soon as someone said they used marijuana, doctors would automatically document a diagnosis of "cannabis abuse." Yes, "abuse" was actually sanctioned as a diagnostic term. These days, I'm happy to report "abuse" has been retired, and more and more healthcare professionals are being trained to evaluate the diagnostic criteria before making a diagnosis of substance use disorder, mild, moderate, or severe.

What You Used to Say:
"This is an example of substance abuse."

What You'll Say Going Forward:
"This is an example of substance use."

Now that we've established the difference between an illness and a crime, let's talk about the difference between use that leads to harm and use that is harmless. Let's start with what might be a controversial statement: not everyone who uses a substance misuses a substance or has a substance use disorder.

It's incredibly important to draw the distinction between substance use, substance misuse, and substance use disorder. To make this as relatable as possible, let's look at drinking alcohol. Nearly 70 percent of American adults drank alcohol in the past year. But only 11.3 percent

INTRODUCTION

of American adults have an alcohol use disorder. Not everyone who drinks would stand up in an AA meeting and say, "I'm an alcoholic." Nor would it be accurate for most of them if they did. However, when we talk about the roughly 48 million Americans who smoke marijuana every year, many people might automatically label them all "potheads." First, let's go ahead and put "pothead" on the list of things we used to say but don't any longer. Second, data suggests that only 10 percent of those who use marijuana will develop an addiction to it. Other research shows that number at 30 percent, meaning an estimated 3 out of 10 regular marijuana users will meet criteria for marijuana use disorder.

Substance use is the rule, not the exception, in America. Think about all the people you encounter in a day and count how many don't do any drugs at all (and yes, alcohol is a drug). Unless you're living in sobriety and have surrounded yourself with people who don't use, the number is probably zero. You bump into your neighbor who does cocaine but only when he's on a boys' weekend in Vegas. You have that friend who admitted to you that she microdosed mushrooms one time and didn't like it. (Or did she?) Most substance use is actually normal behavior. And to label it otherwise contributes to stigma. We're causing people to feel shame and guilt over normal behaviors that don't meet the criteria for "abuse" or a "disorder." It makes it easier for laws like prohibition in the past and the criminalization of marijuana use in the present to exist. Mislabeling substance abuse is also harmful because it puts your health at risk. If you worry that telling your doctor you tried Ambien once is going to make her look at you differently or start talking about getting you into a program, you won't say anything

INTRODUCTION

at all. In fact, research shows that up to 81 percent of people have withheld information from their doctor for a variety of reasons including embarrassment or judgment. One survey found that one of the most common lies patients tell their doctors is around mental health, but drinking, drug use, and smoking are not far behind. That means that the people who you should be comfortable sharing your complete health history with will only have part of the picture, which makes it harder to help. That brings me to another set of confused phrases I'd love to clarify.

What You Used to Say:
"Addict"

What You'll Say Going Forward:
"Person with addiction" or "Person who uses drugs"

If you're not used to people-first language, it might seem a little awkward to get these words out. It may seem much easier to just call someone an "addict." But the problem is that there is tremendous judgment in that phrase. In and of itself it feels like a ruling has been passed down, sentence given, and no possibility for redemption. It makes it seem as if the person is the illness, or that having an addiction is the singular, most important thing about them—which, of course, is never the case.

When we are onboarding staff at Eleanor Health, the company I cofounded, we tell staff flat out, "I don't ever want to hear you call a person an addict." They're a person first, with a condition second. Just as you might mention that your friend Akiba has diabetes or your

INTRODUCTION

friend Jose has asthma, your coworker Natalie may use drugs or have an addiction or be in recovery.

What You Used to Say:
"Drug of choice"

What You'll Say Going Forward:
"Main drug they use" or "Drug they're addicted to"

From a biological perspective, a person with an addiction is someone who continues to use substances even though there are negative physical, mental, social, cultural, and legal consequences tied to that behavior. You've lived long enough and read far enough in this book to know that addiction is not a choice anyone wants to make. No one would choose to lose their job, lose their connection to their loved ones, or harm their own physical or mental health. People in recovery will tell you that while they chose to start using a drug, once their use evolved into a disorder, it was no longer a choice. When we use the term "drug of choice," it implies that a person chose to develop an addiction to that drug. In reality, the compulsion to use the substance was a neurobiological reaction in their brain. The drug, it turns out, chose them.

What You Used to Say:
"He relapsed."

What You'll Say Going Forward:
"His substance use disorder relapsed."

INTRODUCTION

Simply put, people don't relapse. Illnesses relapse. If you had a dear friend who battled lung cancer, it went into remission but then she started smoking again and it came back, you wouldn't say, "She relapsed." That puts the blame on her, not the lung cancer. You'd say, "The cancer came back." So why wouldn't it be the same for someone with a substance use disorder?

The judgment and alienation we put on people with addiction is so clear when we look at how we talk about the recurrence of the disease.

What You Used to Say:
"Relapse is part of the illness."

What You'll Say Going Forward:
"Seventy-five percent of people with substance use disorder recover."

Actually and factually, this is accurate. Relapses occur—just as they do with other types of illnesses. Depending on the stage of colorectal cancer, relapse rates are between 7 and 42 percent in the first five years with a higher relapse rate associated with higher stage at time of diagnosis. But do we tell people with colorectal cancer to expect a recurrence? Do we shrug and whisper behind their backs that relapse is part of the disease? No, we don't. Because that's mean. It's a hope stealer. Because that lacks compassion. It tears someone down instead of building them up.

I don't want to gloss over any fact. Roughly two-thirds (see second chart on page 25) of people in recovery experience a relapse of their

INTRODUCTION

substance use disorder within the first weeks or months of treatment. But as I share that fact with my patients, I focus on the positive. Rather than saying, "Relapse is part of the disease," which makes it seem inevitable, I say, "Two-thirds of people with a substance use disorder will experience a relapse in the first months. Let's talk about the factors that contribute to that and how we try to prevent those factors." The idea is to help drive belief that it is possible for them to be in the group that doesn't experience a relapse. It's time to let go of the negative word-traps and focus on what can happen in that space when we use all our tools to beat addiction.

It's only when we shift the language that we use to discuss addiction, increase the amount of compassion we show to those struggling with addiction, and change the way we think about addiction that we begin to truly care for people with addiction—and reduce our susceptibility to it—forever. So, let's get started.

PART I

The Addiction Risks We Inherit

CHAPTER ONE

Why Some Monkeys Can't Lay Off the Mojitos

The surprising ways DNA impacts the biological risk of substance use

On the undulating sand beaches of St. Kitts, vacationers would prefer to kick back and relax by the water in a Caribbean paradise. Instead, they have to keep their eyes on their drinks—or at least they should if they don't want them stolen. Over the centuries, the island's vervet monkey population has developed an interest in alcohol. It all started with sugarcane stalks being left fermenting in the fields by workers—and then snatched up as a treat by the monkeys. These days, it's transformed into a taste for whatever cocktail the local beach bartender has whipped up.

As soon as beachgoers close their eyes to soak in the sun or abandon their drinks for a dip in the ocean, you'll start to see the one- to two-foot-tall mammals scamper from tree limb to tree limb and then run across the beach to the nearest cup. They'll dunk their whole head into a small glass or simply pick up a cup by its rim and scurry back to the forest while trying not to spill it. Some will even knock over a glass or bottle and lap up what dribbles onto the table.

The aftermath of these stealth tactics is almost as surprising as their scheming to get their little fingers on a Kittian Cowboy or a Ting with a Sting. The boozing monkeys will get fall-down drunk, stumbling as close as they can to home and then passing out on the ground. They'll get into fights over the last sip of margarita left in a cup. They'll shove other monkeys out of the way to try to grab hold of that rum punch.

But not all vervet monkeys drink. And not all vervets drink the same way. When researchers followed 1,000 vervets to understand this fermented phenomenon, they found something interesting about the monkeys' biological predispositions. They discovered that some vervets are social drinkers who sip only after a certain time of day and only with other monkeys. Others are regular imbibers. And still others are teetotalers that would rather knock over a cup of Coke than a bottle of beer to lick up what remains. And finally, about 5 percent are binge drinkers, sadly capable of drinking themselves to death.

So, what do these little critters have to do with me? Over the years, I have worked for public safety net hospitals, nonprofit organizations, and private for-profit mental health companies as the psychiatrist on their addiction treatment team. After my addiction treatment patients have had a comprehensive evaluation with a therapist and are referred to the type of program that would support them the best, they are sent for a psychiatric evaluation with me.

Part of that evaluation involves me determining what that person's concept of themselves is. It may surprise you to hear that people who have struggled with addiction tend to have a negative self-concept.

WHY SOME MONKEYS CAN'T LAY OFF THE MOJITOS

They have had it poured into them that they're terrible, no good, and will never amount to anything. Those are the messages they're getting not just from society but from parents, siblings, spouses, and other loved ones as well. It means they have an overwhelming sense of guilt and moral failure. So, after a certain point in our evaluation, I turn to them and say, "Let me tell you about these monkeys."

We watch a video of the vervets scampering around the beach to grab a cocktail here or a bottle of beer there. We smile. We laugh. And then I say to them, "Can you believe that drunk monkey doesn't care about its family or its friends? That monkey really sucks. It's making terrible choices. Humans would never do that."

And they'll reply, "Actually, that monkey is acting just like me."

And it's true. Vervets behave a lot like humans because we share the majority of our DNA with them. Just like the vervets, we have teetotalers in our midst, and we have binge drinkers among us. We're no different than those monkeys when it comes to alcohol. Instead of scampering across a beach, we're the teenager waiting until her parents fall asleep to sip some vodka and refill the bottle with water. We're the guys getting wasted, stumbling out of a bar and then picking a fight with the first person we see. Just like those drunk monkeys, people who develop an addiction to substances will "choose" drugs or alcohol over food, family, and themselves.

Then I ask my patients to consider an alternative: "What if that monkey's DNA wasn't stacked against him? What if he wasn't in the 5 percent that was likely to drink themselves to death and instead in the teetotaler percentage that had a taste for Fanta instead? What if that monkey had been born on some different island where there were no vacationers or none that left cups of booze all around? What if instead of feeling good, alcohol made their skin turn pink and made them feel overheated? Would they still be drinking like this?"

We go from laughing to being serious. Because it's much harder to give yourself negative messages about being a failure when you see how the odds have been stacked against you. When you're looking at how your biology and your environment impact your addiction risk, suddenly things start to change.

Why People with Addictions Can't Just Make a Different Choice

Despite our exposure to addiction, there's a serious lack of knowledge around this chronic medical condition. Research can offer that knowledge, but only if you happen to read complex medical journals and go to medical conferences like I do. So, I'll break it down for you. The Heritability of Chronic Illnesses chart (see page 25) tells a story that many of us don't get to hear. That addiction can be more easily inherited than asthma, diabetes, hypertension, or breast cancer.

On the left side of the chart is a list of chronic illnesses, which the Centers for Disease Control and Prevention defines as ongoing health conditions (like Alzheimer's, heart disease, or chronic kidney disease) that last a year or more and require long-term medical attention, limit daily activities—or both. They affect the majority of Americans with 60 percent of adults having a chronic illness and about 40 percent having two or more.

WHY SOME MONKEYS CAN'T LAY OFF THE MOJITOS

On the right side of the chart is a list describing how heritable each chronic illness is. Heritability is ranked from zero to one and explains how much your genes account for traits and risks for chronic illnesses. The closer you are to one, the more your risk for developing that illness is coded in your genes. The closer you are to zero, the more the risk is tied to environment or life experiences. So, for example, 34 to 61 percent of your risk of developing addiction is coded in your DNA the day you are born. (For simplicity's sake, let's say that 40 to 60 percent of your addiction risk is inherited.) We also know that the environment and your life experiences make up the remaining 39 to 66 percent. (So, I tell people that 40 to 60 percent of their addiction risk is linked to where they grew up and the life experiences they've had.) Looking at those numbers, you can see that it's pretty hard to "make a different choice" when it's actually addiction that "chooses" you, based on your DNA and the environment you happened to grow up in.

What's important to take away here is that addiction is passed along in our genes like so many other illnesses that we have an overwhelming amount of compassion for, like diabetes and asthma. We vigilantly carry inhalers and watch out for people with breathing conditions. We adjust family dinners and suggest working out together when a loved one has high blood sugar. But for some reason, even though it is also a chronic illness, we treat addiction like a moral failure or a weakness. We look at people who have addiction as individuals we should have contempt for instead of compassion for. We accuse people of choosing to be addicted to substances. But none of us would choose addiction any more than we would choose cancer, diabetes, or asthma.

UN-ADDICTION

One of the ways that researchers look at the heritability of a disease is by examining how frequently the disease appears in identical twins (one fertilized egg that splits) compared to fraternal twins (two eggs separately fertilized) or non-twin siblings. You can't get any closer to deep biological analysis than looking at identical twins: two people who are a DNA carbon copy of each other. If they're raised in different environments, even better because researchers can now see the impact of different parental structures or home settings. As a result, analyzed data shows us not only what the likelihood is of inheriting certain chronic illnesses based on your genes, but also the success in terms of treating those illnesses (see first chart on page 25).

It should also be noted that research has found different addictions are associated with different genes. And while any type of addiction in your family increases your risk of developing addiction in general, it is also the case that *specific* addictions in your family increase your risk of developing that *specific* addiction much more. So, if your mother struggles with alcoholism, your risk for developing any addiction is elevated, but you are particularly at a higher risk for developing alcoholism, as opposed to an addiction to cocaine or marijuana.

The second chart on page 25, about treatment, deserves some special attention. As I mentioned earlier, 30 percent of Americans believe recovery from drug addiction is impossible. "Why bother with going into treatment or detoxing?" they say. "None of it works." But you now know that the one-year relapse rates for addiction are the same as *or lower than* relapse rates for hypertension or asthma. That there's a greater chance of your blood pressure or breathing being out of control than your drug use. For example, studies show that less than 40 percent

Heritability of Chronic Illnesses

ILLNESS	HERITABILITY
Addiction	0.34–0.61
Adult Asthma	0.36–0.70
Type 1 Diabetes	0.30–0.55
Hypertension	0.25–0.50

Relapse Rate of Chronic Illnesses

ILLNESS	FOLLOWS TREATMENT RECOMMENDATIONS	RELAPSE RATE (1 YR)
Addiction	40–60%	40–60%
Asthma	<40% meds <30% lifestyle	>60%
Diabetes	<60% meds <30% lifestyle	30–50%
Hypertension	<40% meds <30% lifestyle	50–70%

Source: McLellan AT, Lewis DC, O'Brien CP, Kleber HD. "Drug dependence, a chronic medical illness: implications for treatment, insurance, and outcomes evaluation." *JAMA*. 2000 Oct 4;284(13):1689-95. doi: 10.1001/jama.284.13.1689.

of adults with asthma stick to their recommended medication schedule. Do you wonder, "Why can't they just make a different choice?" No. And yet, that is what we are saying to people who are struggling with addiction.

So much of the work that I do as a specialist in addiction medicine has to do with unpacking and rewriting the narrative that many of us have adhered to for a long time. Here are the false truths I hear again and again:

UN-ADDICTION

False Truths:
- ❯ People with active addiction can just decide to stop using substances if they really want to.

- ❯ They don't want to be contributing members of society.

- ❯ They don't care about the impact of their behavior.

- ❯ They are bad people because they struggle with substance use.

- ❯ Addiction is a lifestyle choice that gets handed down through families.

Newer, Truer Narrative:
- ❯ When you look at the research, 40 to 60 percent of your risk is passed on to you the day you are born.

- ❯ Having a parent who is dependent on alcohol can biologically impact you, resulting in you having a higher tolerance and potentially drinking more.

- ❯ Addiction isn't a lifestyle choice but a biological imperative (think: survival instinct, like procreation) that gets handed down through families through DNA.

- ❯ People with active addiction frequently don't get the support that they need to understand what's happening to them and how they can change it.

WHY SOME MONKEYS CAN'T LAY OFF THE MOJITOS

The good news here is that if 40 to 60 percent of our risk is out of our control, the same percentage is actually within our control. But what exactly do we have to do to take that control back?

You can't ask someone to save a plane from crashing without teaching them how to fly. You can't ask someone to not eat when they're starving. And you can't simply "make a different choice" when your biological imperative is telling you to choose the drug (alcohol included) and your environment makes the drug the easier, if not the only, choice. Though we know our addiction risk is coded into our DNA, that's exactly what we're asking people who struggle with substance use disorders to do when we don't give them the knowledge and tools to heal. What's worse, we make it even harder for them to recover by robbing them of compassion, hope, and the kind of emotional support any person needs when they are suffering.

Throughout my career, I've seen the transformational impact that compassion can have on someone who struggles with substance use. I think about the mom who came to me ready to throw her teenager out onto the street after discovering a baggie with white powder in his room while cleaning up. She had just lost her husband (his father) and was on the verge of letting go of her son. By changing her approach from "You can't live here anymore" to "You can't use drugs in this house and here are the new random drug testing rules for our home," instead of losing a son (and potentially a daughter, who had sympathy for her brother) she and her children actually got closer and the usage stopped.

I also think about the grandmother who was babysitting her granddaughter when she fell asleep while smoking crack in bed. The mattress caught fire and she came frighteningly close to the kind of mistake that would be terrifying to live with. The baby could've died. The house could have burned down. Everyone inside could have perished. I worked with that grandmother and her estranged daughter for over a year. At the eighteen-month mark, we had a celebration of sobriety and that grandmother showed up with her daughter—and her granddaughter. Their reunion brought tears to my eyes.

Now, let's be clear. I'm not saying addiction is an illness just to make you feel better about struggling with it or to try to pry some compassion out of you for loved ones who are struggling with it. I'm telling you addiction is an illness because that is a fact.

When I work with my patients, their loved ones, and now, with you, I'm like a prosecutor presenting my case in front of a jury. Many people have been inculcated with the belief that their loved ones struggling with substance use are just bad people. How could you not? Some of my patients and their loved ones have had horrible misfortunes because of their active addiction. How could that grandmother with the burned bed not feel terrible? Then again—she is sick. She wasn't in her right mind. If she were in her right mind, smoking crack with her grandbaby nearby isn't a choice she would have made. Once we understand the biological power that drugs have over our thoughts, feelings, emotions, decisions, and behavior, then we can assign the blame and point our contempt to the addiction, rather than to the person. So, let's talk about why drugs have that power over us.

The Four Parts of the Brain Associated with Addiction

It's time for a quick—but critical—neurobiology lesson. Hang in there with me! First, let's talk about your limbic system. It's a series of structures

WHY SOME MONKEYS CAN'T LAY OFF THE MOJITOS

and connections in our brains that are responsible for our thoughts, emotions, reactions, and behavior. Your **amygdala** (think: emotions), an almond-shaped structure in your brain, is part of that system. It's specifically responsible for assigning emotional memory to experiences. Fight or flight goes through the amygdala. It can make you feel uncertainty, sadness, depression, fear, and more—and it sends those messages to the prefrontal cortex. We'll talk more about the prefrontal cortex in a second, but first let's talk about the dopamine pathway.

When you think of your **dopamine pathway**, think needs. Also known as "The Motivation Pathway" or "The Reward Pathway," it is committed to your survival. It makes sure we continue to do those things that will keep us alive (as individuals and as a species). From an evolutionary perspective, it tells us what we need: Food. Water. Sex. Nurturing. It starts deep in the brain and is made up of three neurons that pass messages along, one by one, until that message also lands on the prefrontal cortex.

Finally, there's your **prefrontal cortex** (think: reactions). It's designed to react without you having to make decisions because everything is a matter of survival. It's how a race car driver can drive 200 miles per hour and turn corners. It's how Sully Sullenberger could land that plane on the Hudson River. His full-body feeling from his amygdala might have been panic, but his prefrontal cortex was trained to react otherwise.

Now let's take things back a few thousand years to the prehistoric age, where we're just trying to survive in the jungle in our coconut bras and loincloths. You're sitting by a warm fire when you hear something rustling in the bushes. You know that footfall. It's probably a gazelle that could be perfect to cook on that fire. Your stomach starts to growl as you imagine something amazing for dinner.

"I'm excited. It's been three days since we had anything to eat," says your amygdala (emotions).

"We're starving. Let's make a plan to eat that gazelle," says your dopamine pathway (needs).

"I've got a plan for killing that gazelle," says your prefrontal cortex (reactions), as adrenaline starts to rush in. "Let's go quietly gather some rocks."

"I'm getting more excited," says your amygdala. "I remember the last time we ate gazelle, it was off the chain. We were starving and it felt like the life came back into us."

"This is perfect," says your dopamine pathway. "Food will keep us alive and propagate the species. Let's plan to never go without gazelle meat again."

Sound about right? In fact, it probably sounds harmless and critical to survival. Until I ask you to swap out the gazelle . . . for cocaine. Or marijuana. Or a glass of Chardonnay. Instead of being a protein-rich gazelle, it could be a substance that also *feels* like it gives you life and feeds you but can lead to addiction.

And what's worse, while food and sex are incredibly strong stimuli for your brain, they're nothing compared to drugs. If the allure of food to a hungry person is a candle, drugs would be the blazing hot intensity of a thousand suns in comparison. Biologically, crack, meth, heroin, alcohol, marijuana, and cigarettes are more important than food, sex, water, and family, purely because of the size of the dopamine signal they can generate.

Finally, this back-and-forth dialogue takes less than a second. And even though your limbic and dopamine systems' reactions are

WHY SOME MONKEYS CAN'T LAY OFF THE MOJITOS

instantaneous, your prefrontal cortex can still claim a fraction of a second to make a different choice. Whenever you have an experience that naturally triggers a dopamine signal (think stimuli like delicious food, water, great sex, nurturing, or drugs), you don't have to succumb to it. Even though your amygdala might be saying, "This is a dangerous situation, let's put on a parachute and get out of here!" or the dopamine pathway may be telling your prefrontal cortex, "You need this pizza/three-way/cocaine to survive! Make a plan for us to never go without it," you still have time to question that message before taking action.

In addiction rehab, we train your prefrontal cortex not to immediately believe everything that the limbic system is telling it. Even though your brain can get hijacked by legal and illegal substances, it's possible to remind it that drugs are not more important than other elements of your life. We show patients how to question its authority and not take that information as gold. When your prefrontal cortex says, "Let's go get that gazelle/cocaine, or else!" you can respond, "Or else what? We're not going to survive? I don't think so." We teach patients how to take a different set of circumstances into account. "Actually," they realize, "if I *get* that drug, I might *not* survive."

And you know what the best part is? You don't have to wait until you need rehab to train your prefrontal cortex to question your limbic and dopamine systems. There are so many simple, small things any of us can do to buy our prefrontal cortex some time to make a better decision. Engaging in just five minutes of deep breathing or mindfulness meditation practice can lower your blood pressure, decrease your heart rate, and improve your concentration. All of those biological changes increase your prefrontal cortex's ability to think clearly and make healthy decisions. Too much of a commitment? How about just promising yourself you'll count to ten before getting up to go to the kitchen or type your credit card number into the website?

Another great option is to adopt a mantra that you repeat in difficult situations like, "Think first! Think first! Think first!" Or try a visualization exercise recommended by Alcoholics Anonymous (AA) where you "play the tape until the end." You're basically imagining yourself in a movie and asking yourself, "If I make this decision now, what happens next? And after that?" until you get to the end of this movie. Both exercises not only create some space between the physical *reaction* that your body is having and the physical *action* you're about to take—they're also allowing you to take time to consider the consequences of that action and make a different decision. While you're "thinking first" and "playing the tape," you might worry about driving home high, having nonconsensual sex, upsetting your partner by coming to bed smelling of smoke, waking up hungover, getting to work late, losing your job, and so on. The beauty of these techniques is that they help you avoid making unhealthy choices on autopilot.

Preventing Addiction in Yourself: Family History Awareness

You've probably heard people say that the first step to solving a problem is recognizing that you have one. But with substance use, the very first step to preventing a problem can happen even sooner, by recognizing a family history of problems. Awareness of your family history is part of the Magic Formula™ for empowering yourself to reduce your risk of developing addiction.

Long before you get invited to a high school kegger, get handed your first Xanax, or are offered your first bump of cocaine, you need to be aware of how those substances can impact you. I don't mean in the generic "Just Say No" sense. I'm talking about your personalized risk for developing an addiction based on your biology.

While that may sound extreme to you now, I doubt you'd consider it unreasonable for other biologically inherited health concerns. How many times have you filled out an intake form at a doctor's office and written down the people in your family that have had heart attacks or cancer? You can do that very same work to figure out what substance use disorders you may be at increased risk for due to your DNA.

Remember, it's not just addiction in general, but also an increased risk for addiction to specific substances that can run in a family. People in your family might be more likely to inherit a vulnerability to chaotic use of opioids and alcohol while your friend might inherit an increased risk for amphetamines or cigarettes from their family. The same way that a woman might get tested for the BRCA gene because breast cancer runs in her family, a person can analyze their biological risk for addictive problems in general—as well as for specific types.

Getting a handle on your family history looks like asking yourself two simple questions.

Question #1: *Is there anyone in my family that people thought had a problem with substance use?*

This isn't the time to overlook that grandmother who was tipsy all the time or to start rationalizing how your uncle was never the same after going into the Army. Of course, I want you to be compassionate. But the goal of asking yourself this question isn't to judge others but to look at some basic facts and determine what they mean for your biological risk. This also isn't the time to disregard certain types of substance use. Cigarettes, cigars, chewing tobacco, and vaping all count. Even though it may be more socially acceptable than marijuana or opioids, nicotine is a highly addictive substance and is so readily available, which makes it even more difficult to quit. Nicotine runs through the same dopamine pathway as all the other drugs of addiction.

Question #2: *Has anyone in my family outwardly struggled with substance use?*

If you answered yes to this question, then you have an increased biological risk for addiction. But there's no need to panic. In fact, the opposite. Despite what you may have heard, there are real, concrete steps you can take to reduce your risk of developing an addiction. Being educated on your biological risk means you can use that information to make different decisions out of the gate. If you know that several women in your family have had breast cancer, chances are you're less likely to smoke that first cigarette. You might even get more vegetables in your diet and start up a yoga practice just in case. You may be more motivated to remember your monthly breast exam. Well, if you know several people in your immediate family struggle with substance use, you can make similar decisions to decrease your risk. You can choose to avoid first exposure to addictive substances. You can decide to explore healthy habits for dealing with stress so you're not compelled to turn to substances as a way to cope. You can talk to your kids about their risk and practice an ounce of generational prevention.

One smart way to track this information is by creating an addiction family tree (see pages 238–239). Instead of names or pictures for each branch of your family, like you'd have in a regular family tree, you can jot down whether or not there was a substance use concern. For a tree like this, I recommend mapping out three generations, which includes your grandparents, parents, aunts, and uncles, plus you and your siblings. As you fill out each branch, you may start to notice trends in the number of relatives who struggled with substance use and the types of substances they used.

After family history, the second level of awareness you need to prevent substance use disorders is an awareness of its early warning signs.

Diagnosing Addiction in Yourself: Behavioral Awareness

Preachers and pastors rely on the Bible as their source of truth. The diagnostic bible for psychiatrists, clinical psychologists, and other behavioral health professionals is a 1,000-page book put out by the American Psychiatric Association called the *Diagnostic and Statistical Manual of Mental Disorders: 5th Edition.* (Or the DSM-V for short.) Every updated edition of the DSM is an evolution in medicine that names and offers criteria for new and existing mental health disorders. The most recent edition of the DSM made a huge step in the right direction to help understand addiction. Previously, it presented an outdated concept of addiction that offered only two categories for substance use disorder: substance abuse and substance dependence. It inherently drove stigma by driving professional use of the term "abuse." In the current edition, the DSM expanded and renamed the possibilities to include three categories of substance use disorders: mild, moderate, and severe. I'll tell you why this is such a huge deal in a moment, but first let's talk about how to figure out if you fall into one of those three categories.

The DSM-V includes a list of eleven criteria to evaluate a possible diagnosis of substance use disorder. You might be asked if you had times, in the past year, when you wanted to use a substance so badly you couldn't think of anything else. Or if you had gotten into situations while using that substance that increased your odds of getting hurt. That could be drinking and driving or having unsafe sex. You might even be asked if you ever ended up indulging in the substance more than you wanted to or found that using it interfered with taking care of your home or family.

If you answer "yes" to six or more of these criteria, then you qualify as having a severe substance use disorder. But what if you score less than six? Does that mean you don't have anything to worry about? Is the world only made of up people with severe addiction calling in sick for work because they're hungover and those who are functioning perfectly fine using substances? Not a chance. If you answer "yes" to two or three criteria, that signals a mild disorder. Four or five means a moderate disorder. These mild and moderate categories are now being called "preaddiction"—a concept I wish I'd come up with because it has the power to change everything. Let me tell you why.

WHY SOME MONKEYS CAN'T LAY OFF THE MOJITOS

Up until about two decades ago, the medical world put people in two categories: those with diabetes and those without diabetes. Then the term "prediabetes" was coined around 2003 to drive early intervention. Experts wanted to recognize the signs of an increased risk for diabetes and decrease the number of people who progressed to the full disease with lifestyle, dietary, and medical efforts. And some would say it was a huge success. There has been a 35 percent decrease in cases of diagnosed diabetes since rates peaked in 2009. The question now is, could the same happen for addiction?

There's a lot to love about this new word: "preaddiction." First, the term "preaddiction" has the ability to reduce fear and stigma—two of the biggest obstacles that prevent people from getting support or help after getting sick. It's much less terrifying to tell a family member or lover that you have "precancerous" cells on your cervix versus saying you have cervical cancer. The same emotional impact applies to preaddiction.

Second, a severe addiction doesn't usually happen overnight. It most often takes years to develop as a person progresses from mild to moderate to severe use.

For decades, most of the medical community was waiting for people to hit "rock bottom" in their severe addiction to take action. But why not try to prevent rock bottom, especially when research shows that a brief intervention with your doctor (just a *two-minute* discussion) about your addictive concerns can change your behavior? That's right, I said, *just two minutes*. Having a term like "preaddiction" functions as a wake-up call and encourages efforts to get help before the person and their family are in crisis. What's beautiful about the work we do at Eleanor Health is that we've always embraced that. You don't have to say, "I have an addiction" to get help. We open our doors in several ways to people experiencing various levels of addiction, including preaddiction, which empowers more people to stop the progression of the illness.

By now you're probably wondering, "If these eleven questions are so great, why won't Nzinga tell us what they are right here?" Because the average person doesn't need all eleven questions to figure out their risk. You can actually just start with four. In addiction medicine, there's another very easy tool for identifying early warning signs for addiction called CAGE. It's a series of questions you can ask yourself to figure out how concerned you should be about your substance use. The acronym unfolds like this:

C: "Have I ever thought I should **CUT** back on my drinking/vaping/cocaine use/etc.?"

A: "Have I ever felt **ANNOYED** when someone said to me, 'Do you think you should cut back on your drinking/vaping/cocaine use/etc.?'?"

G: "Have you ever felt **GUILTY** because you said, 'I'm only going to have one glass of wine tonight' or 'I'm not going to vape today' but then made it to your third glass or picked up the pen anyway?" Or maybe when you go to your annual physical and your doctor asks if you smoke, drink, or do drugs, you get the impetus to minimize it. Or just flat out keep it hush-hush. You might also feel this on occasions when you've drunk more or used more than you meant to. Or if you've ever felt that you wanted to cut down on your drinking or drug use.

E: "Have you ever relied on a substance as an **EYE-OPENER**?" That means first thing in the morning, after you wake up and open your eyes, you're thinking about vaping or drinking. Or you actually go vape or have a drink.

Roughly 80 percent of the time, a "yes" answer to any one of these questions represents a substance use disorder, whether mild, moderate, or severe. The other 20 percent of the time, a "yes" answer to any of these questions represents a risk you now have the power to reduce.

If there's one thing I want you to do after reading that list of questions and getting even a single "yes," it's to accept that your use is risky without judging yourself. It's that judgment, that silence, that guilt that holds so many of us back from seeking help. And a "yes" to any of those CAGE questions should be a signal to you that it's time to seek help. Do not pass go, do not collect $200, reach out for help as soon as possible.

If you had prediabetes, your doctor might recommend adopting the Mediterranean diet and making sure to get 10,000 steps in a day, among other strategies. For preaddiction, I've come up with the following Magic Formula™ for success.

Step One: *Don't hesitate. Reach out for help immediately.*

We all need one person that we can talk to specifically about our alcohol or drug use. The whole point is not to keep your new knowledge in the dark. You can pick a trusted friend, a primary care doctor, your partner, your therapist, your gynecologist, a religious/spiritual guide, a support group on the web. There's no shortage of people I want you to think of reaching out to. The goal is not to hide the fact that you're worried about your substance use. You have to tell at least one other person if you want to reduce the chance your concerns ever become catastrophic. It's not a bad idea to prepare yourself for a variety of reactions. Your best friend may, in turn, tell you about her use of sedatives. Your doctor might be caught off guard and need time to do some research before coming back to you with recommendations.

Step Two: *Cut your use in half.*

Instead of cutting down on sodium (for hypertension) or carbs (for diabetes), you're going to be cutting back on drinking, smoking, snorting, or inhaling. And you're going to do it by 50 percent in a week's time. Anyone who reduces their risk by half significantly reduces the impact of a substance on their physical and mental health. The problem is most people don't know exactly how much they're using a substance to begin with. (There goes that key factor of awareness again.) You can start keeping track using the Substance Use Journal template, which I've included on page 240, or your own journal. If you use your own, at a minimum, be sure to record the date, day of the week, time, what you used, how much you used, how you were feeling before you used it, who you were with, and what you were doing.

All these details provide insight into your use patterns. You might realize, *I'm drinking because I'm sad* or *I'm vaping marijuana to relax as soon as the kids fall asleep* or *I'm drinking to fall asleep* or *I only smoke after arguing with my partner* or *When I hang out with this person, that's when I do heroin.* That gives you a place to start a use pattern change. Maybe you stop hanging out with your heroin partner. Perhaps you call a friend when you start to feel sad. Bringing your behavior to consciousness means your prefrontal cortex can start making different decisions. The alternative is operating on autopilot. And when substances are involved, autopilot is the fast track to severe illness.

WHY SOME MONKEYS CAN'T LAY OFF THE MOJITOS

If you're not able to cut your use in half, get professional help immediately. If you are, try cutting it in half one more time to truly get things under control.

Step Three: *Retake the CAGE questionnaire.*

After a week of trying to cut back by half, ask yourself the four CAGE questions again but make them specific to the past seven days.

C: "In the past week of journaling, did I ever think I should **cut** back?"

A: "In the past week of journaling, did I feel increasingly **annoyed** by criticisms of my substance use?"

G: "In the past week of journaling, have I felt **guilty** about my substance use?"

E: "In the past week of journaling, did I need an **eye-opener** in the morning?"

If you still answer "yes" to even one of these questions, it's time to get professional help.

Step Four: *Talk to your PCP.*

You don't have to trudge all the way down to your doctor's office, but at the very least book an e-visit with your primary care physician to let them know what's going on. You might say, "I read some new research about preaddiction and I am worried about my substance use. What are some things I can do to avoid addiction?" Or "I just took the CAGE test and I've been keeping a Substance Use Journal for the past few weeks because I'm concerned about my substance use. What can I do to protect myself?" Don't be surprised if you must educate your doctor on what the CAGE test is or what preaddiction is. But do give them time to take it all in and get back to you with helpful answers around prevention.

Step Five: *Download tech support.*
Take this as an opportunity to lean on technology to get your desired outcome of decreasing your risk. There are a ton of free apps on the market that can help you feel more empowered, get more information in the moment, and see the impact of your new choices as you decrease or eliminate your substance use. See pages 236–237 for suggestions. You might also check out apps that help people with stress, anxiety, and depression, which may increase as you decrease your substance use. Take the opportunity to get support no matter where you are so long as you have your phone with you.

Mind-Changing Conversation #1: Talks That Can Prevent Addiction in Your Loved Ones

The idea that we can't talk about addiction is what keeps addiction going. But when we create environments where loved ones can come talk to us if they recognize the signs of addiction in themselves, we can stop addiction in its tracks. Now that you have a baseline understanding of how to think about genetic risk for addiction in yourself, you can imagine how you might want someone to approach you or support you if they were worried about you struggling with a substance. Once you've decided to reach out to a loved one about their struggle—and you should reach out—follow one of my checklists for making sure you hit every necessary note of that conversation.

Checklist for Family Member or Friend

Get crystal clear on what's a problem. Substance use is not one size fits all. The National Institute on Alcohol Abuse and Alcoholism defines heavy drinking as three drinks on any day or more than seven drinks per week for women and four drinks on any day or more than fourteen drinks per week for a man. But we all know people who are buzzed after one glass of champagne or seem to be able to drink everyone else at the party under the table. You and your family member or friend are going to have to talk about what constitutes a problem.

It might sound something like: "I'm worried about you, and I need to figure out how I will know if your substance use is a problem. What would realistic red flags look like?"

Ending up under a bridge with all your possessions in a shopping cart is not the answer, but that's often immediately where people's minds go. The two of you are going to set those boundaries and red flags together in your conversation. This is what practicing an ounce of prevention looks like. Some people may happily set a boundary of only smoking marijuana on the weekend and recognize that smoking during the week is an early warning sign.

Let the conversation lean on the numbers. Numbers don't lie, so if you're already concerned about their substance use, try to start off the conversation there. Confidently drop the statistic I've already shared with you about how up to 60 percent of addiction is coded in our DNA the day we're born. Then compel them to take responsibility for the other 40 to 60 percent to help themselves and their loved ones. It might sound like: "It's not your fault that you're struggling—or that you don't think you're struggling. But now that we understand the numbers, it's your responsibility to try to get this illness in remission for you and for all the kids in our family that have the same DNA."

Educate yourself on enabling. What changes human behavior is consequences. Enabling a loved one removes the natural consequences of their behavior. We unintentionally enable substance use in many ways—by giving money, by protecting from legal consequences, by making excuses. By removing the natural consequences of a person's behavior, we delay the time it will take for them to realize they need to make a change. Word of caution here, though: avoiding enabling does *not* mean letting someone hit rock bottom. For too many, rock bottom is death—and that is not what any of us want. That leads me right to the next section, which is setting compassionate boundaries.

Set compassionate boundaries for yourself. Be sure you're setting boundaries with your family member or friend and that you're emotionally prepared to maintain those boundaries. Maybe that means they can always visit your house, but they can't stay overnight. Or you'll buy clothes for their children, but never give them a direct loan. It takes a lot of support to do this and can get very difficult, but if you can get everyone in your family on the same page, that will be a good start. Often, getting professional support in place for yourself will help you provide the support you need to your loved one.

WHY SOME MONKEYS CAN'T LAY OFF THE MOJITOS

Checklist for a Partner

Get crystal clear on what's a problem. You and your partner must talk about what constitutes a problem. You'll set those boundaries and red flags together. It might sound something like: "I know that X runs in your family, and I'm worried about you developing the same. I need to figure out how I will know if any substance use becomes a problem."

If you're already seeing behaviors that are making you concerned, then it's time to have a compassionate talk. The first time you think to yourself, *Are they drinking/smoking too much?* the answer is yes. Don't second-guess yourself. Don't downplay the situation. Don't ignore what you're seeing. Trust your intuition and trust what you've seen in other members of your partner's (or your own) family.

Have the conversation in a nonjudgmental way. Let them know that you are doing your best to view their behaviors in a nonjudgmental way and that you're worried about the dangers that their substance use poses. Would they be able to prioritize your health and safety if not for the addiction? Remind them of their inherited risk factors from their family and assure them that you two are in this together. It might sound like this: "I know other people in your family have struggled with substances. I think this is what I'm seeing now. I'm bringing it up because you have a biological risk and I want to stay in front of it. Can the two of us be pointed against addiction together?"

Educate yourself on enabling. What changes human behavior is consequences. Enabling a loved one removes the natural consequences of their behavior. Every time you recycle beer bottles in the dead of night so the kids don't notice or take on more bills because their money is going to drugs, you're eliminating the consequences of their behavior. You're also delaying the time until they realize they need to make a change.

Set compassionate boundaries for yourself. Be sure you're setting boundaries with your partner and that you're emotionally prepared to maintain those boundaries. Maybe that means they do recreational drugs when your kids are away for the weekend. Or you'll never buy alcohol for them, but they can get it on their own. It takes a lot of strength to do this and can get very difficult, but your partner's inability to stick to agreed boundaries around substance use is another signal to you that something has gone wrong.

Get support for yourself. People always think, "I have to get them into treatment!" or "I have to convince them to change!" Every time someone comes to me concerned about a loved one, I tell them: You can control what *you* do but you can't control what *others* do. So, control how you speak to them. Go to a therapist, counselor, or faith leader and say all the ugly things to your therapist unfiltered so you don't say them to your loved one.

Then work with that trusted confidant to figure out how you convey what you need to say in a way that's more effective to your person. When someone in your circle struggles with substances, as we know from flight safety instructions, you have to put the oxygen mask on yourself before you try to put it on them. Get support in place for yourself so you have the education you need about the illness they have.

Checklist for a Child

You might be spending all your energy hiding drugs and alcohol from your three- or four-year-old. Here's your wake-up call: They've already seen it. On the street, on the bus, on television, in the movies. If there's a genetic predisposition for addiction in your family, chances are your child will lay eyes on it at home, too. Don't fool yourself. These kids are watching every move you make, and they notice when something's not quite right. When teachers go around the class at school asking what Daddy's favorite drink is, they say beer, not coffee or lemonade. By the way, that's an early warning sign for how much you're drinking and the perception of drinking your child is developing.

Beyond noticing alcohol and drug use, kids participate in it at early ages as well. The people who come into my office will tell me that their first drink was at age nine or that they started smoking at ten or using heroin at age eleven. I can almost hear some of you saying to yourselves right now, "Not my kid! Not in elementary school." But it could be your kid. I'm trying to make sure it's not your kid right now with this advice.

You don't have to create opportunities to have this conversation. Life is going to bring opportunities to you. Preschool isn't too young to start to have talks with your child about what they've witnessed, how they feel about it, and what it means. But guess what? If you've missed that boat, high school isn't too late, either. These are critical conversations that most of us have never had. But they're capable of changing lives and even saving them. Here are some key talking points to use no matter how old your babies are.

If the child is a preschooler:

Ask, don't tell. When we approach children, we often start with the idea, "Let me tell you something." But we should start with, "Did you see what happened? What did you think of that?" Maybe you know they've noticed their father dumping cigarette butts into the trash. You could ask, "Did you see Daddy put the cigarettes in the garbage? What did you think about that?" They might be angry that Daddy lied about not smoking or disappointed that he broke a promise about not smoking anymore. Whatever they say, validate their emotions and then send them in the direction of understanding and compassion.

Combine compassion with information. You're having this conversation at, perhaps, the one moment in time when your child won't have anger, resentment, or even hatred toward someone in your family who is struggling with addiction. It's extremely important to make sure that you strengthen their compassion muscle while also helping them understand what's happening. To do this, you must separate the illness from the person. That may sound like: "Addiction is an illness but it's not like every other illness. It's not like a cold, because you stop sneezing and coughing after a few days with a cold. It's more like asthma where you have to carry around an inhaler for the rest of your life. You know your friend Jane who gets really sick from asthma and we hate that it keeps her from coming to school or going to parties with you? Addiction is an illness just like asthma, it just starts in the brain instead of the lungs. Addiction runs in our family, and this is how you can tell when a person is struggling."

Differentiate addiction from the person with the addiction. Make sure that your child knows they're upset with the illness and not the person who is sick. You might say, "That's addiction, not your dad." Or "We're mad at addiction, not at Daddy. We care about Daddy and want him to get better."

Make the connection. This is your opportunity to explain to your child how addiction can be passed along biologically. You might say: "Sometimes addiction runs in families. You know how you look like Daddy, and you and I like the same foods? That's because we gave you our DNA! Pretty cool, huh? It also means there are some things we have to look out for—like asthma and addiction—that run in our family. The good news is, because we know all about our DNA, we know how to protect you, and you'll learn how to protect yourself!" Now I know this may seem like a sophisticated conversation to have with a four- or five-year-old, but trust me, they get it.

If the child is in elementary school:

Ask, don't tell. Then draw them in. By this age, almost every single kid knows they have someone at home, or they have a friend with someone at home, who is struggling with addiction. They've also gotten media and cultural messages about alcohol and drug use that inevitably has them thinking: *I can't wait to party with friends and have a drink when I'm eighteen!* or *I can't wait until my friends and I sneak away to try smoking!*

UN-ADDICTION

You want to be inquisitive and make sure that they know they can come to you with any concerns. You want them walking away from your talk with a new message: *Wow! If I'm ever worried about myself or my friends, I can talk to my parents about this. I could really come to them!*

Whenever the opportunity arises at a family cookout, while you're watching TV, or after someone visits your home, your conversation might start something like this: "What do you and your friends think about alcohol/pills/marijuana? Do you guys talk about that? Do you think your friends can talk to their parents about it? You know, you can always talk to me about this. They can too. I would never want you to try anything but if you do and ever think it's becoming risky, you can come and talk to me about that."

Differentiate addiction from the person with the addiction. At this age, kids are focused on black/white, right/wrong thinking. Make sure that your goal here is to educate them about addiction as an illness that is separate from the person they love. The conversation might start something like: "You know, addiction can be tricky. It's an illness, but because the symptoms can be very hurtful, sometimes we can think it's our person we hate, instead of the illness. Even in the hardest times, we have to remind ourselves that the person we love is also suffering, and the illness is the one to blame, not them."

Make the connection. You can be more scientific when you talk to older kids about their risk. Mention DNA and physical illnesses that run in your family. You might say: "You know how everyone in our

WHY SOME MONKEYS CAN'T LAY OFF THE MOJITOS

family has high blood pressure? That's because some of that risk is in our DNA. You know how we're worried about Grandma's alcohol use/cigarette smoking? That means we have risk for that in our DNA, too. So, we need to talk about ways to keep each other safe."

If you have a middle schooler:

Ask, don't tell. Then help them make smart decisions. It's so important for kids this age to feel like they're fitting in. That can make peer pressure public enemy number one or biggest ally number one depending on what their friends think about drug use. So, when you inquire about what they're experiencing, it's important to reinforce that they make the decision that may not be the most popular but certainly is the safest. Your conversation might start out: "What are your and your friends' thoughts on alcohol, cigarettes, pills? Anyone using those? Anyone have access to those? Is it cool? Dangerous?

"You know, what is safe for someone else is not necessarily safe for you because of your DNA. Your friends may be able to take a couple of pills or eat a marijuana brownie and be perfectly fine, but our DNA makes that a bigger risk for you. So, if someone offered you drugs, the safest choice is always to say no.

"But no matter what choice you make, you can always come talk to me if you're worried about yourself or your friends. Or if you have questions. You're not going to get in trouble for bringing me this conversation. You might think it will change the way I feel about you—and it will; that's because I'll be so grateful and know how amazing it is that you came to me."

If the child is a high schooler:

Imagine it has already happened. I need you to get past the head-shaking and that heart-sinking feeling in your stomach because I need you to be calm if and when your child tells you they've used drugs. I want you to close your eyes, take a few deep breaths to stay calm, and then visualize finding a small baggie of something in your kid's pocket as you're doing the laundry. Or coming across an empty bottle while cleaning their room. Then push past that fear, anger, and anxiety so you can keep your cool when you approach them.

Practice the conversation that you'd have with them. Think of it as an opportunity—not a catastrophe. Your kid isn't dead. Your kid isn't in a hospital. You have an opportunity to disrupt their trajectory.

You'll want to use all the skills that I suggested with younger kids: Hammer home that as much as 60 percent of their risk is in their DNA. Make sure they know it's you and them against addiction—not addiction tearing your relationship apart. Reassure them that you trust them to make the safest decision and come to you if they're worried.

But you'll also need to give them some tools, like a "safe word" they can use if they need to call you to jettison them out of a tricky situation—without looking bad to their friends. You might say to your child: "If you find yourself in a difficult situation, call me. I will always come get you—even if you are drunk, even if you're high, even if it's the worst situation you'd never want me to know you're in. I promise you, I'm the safest person for you to call. Dad and I will have our phones by us. You can shoot us a text with a safe word. And then tell your friends, 'My mom said I gotta get home now.'"

WHY SOME MONKEYS CAN'T LAY OFF THE MOJITOS

If your child is already using substances, it's still important to get inquisitive. You might ask: "What are your goals around using? Do you see it as being dangerous? Do you want to use in a non-dangerous way? Are your friends using?"

Know your boundaries. Let your child know that you're on their side, but there are scenarios you will and won't accept. It could be that they can't smoke marijuana in your house, but you'll look the other way if they do it elsewhere. Or you'd rather they drink alcohol safely at home but never bring people in to drink with them. (Either way, you'll want to check the laws in your state before you decide what you will and won't allow your child to do in or out of the home.) It may be that you don't want them smoking or drinking at all—and there will be tests. You can also remind your child of how they've seen addiction impact the lives of those they love in the family. That may not change their choices, but it will help them shift their perspective, and it will plant seeds in the event future intervention becomes necessary.

Un-Addicted: Your Inherited Biological Risk

In this section, I presented my case for biology determining addiction risk. In the next section, I'll show you the psychological factors that tip the scales of addiction. Understanding psychological factors can help us (and our loved ones) reduce our risk of developing addiction and increase our chances of recovery should an addiction develop. We've covered a lot of science so far, though, and I want to remind you of what we've just learned.

Key Takeaways

> **Your risk for addiction is built into your DNA.**
> Addiction is not a choice. After all, who would willingly make that choice to suffer? Instead, genetics determines up to 60 percent of your susceptibility. That means much of your risk of developing an addiction is biologically inherited.

> **Addiction's heritability trumps other chronic illnesses.**
> In some cases, substance use is more likely to be passed on genetically than other ailments such as diabetes, high blood pressure, and asthma. You can't just "snap out" of shortness of breath; and you can't just "snap out" of addiction.

> **Spotting preaddiction can improve addiction rates.**
> Just like prediabetes, prehypertension, precancer, osteopenia, and more, preaddiction is being recognized as a mild to moderate version of its full chronic health condition counterpart, addiction. Recognizing the signs of preaddiction and

acting on them can help you prevent addiction down the line.

> **Knowledge is prevention power.**
Identifying the biological links to addiction in yourself and others can also empower you to be more intentional about prevention. So can knowing the right words to say at the right time.

Your Homework

> **Create an Addiction Family Tree.**
Ask family members about relatives that have struggled with substance use. By tracing which substances were used and by whom, you can assess your risk and the risk of others in your family. (See My Addiction Family Tree on pages 238-239.)

> **Paint an accurate profile.**
When talking with your relatives about loved ones in your family tree who have a substance use disorder, use four to five positive adjectives to describe them in the present tense. Think of them for who they are, not for the disease they have.

> **Break the silence.**
Ask a loved one to talk to you about a family member that no one talks about. Hidden stories in your family are sometimes tied to the shame of substance use. Starting the conversation can stop a cycle of use. Encourage your loved one to share at least five to ten details about your family member

that have nothing to do with substance use so you're able to see them as more than their chronic illness.

> » **Practice honesty with your PCP.**
> When you go in for checkups, fill out your addiction family history truthfully or update your doctor as to what you may have left out in previous visits. Use your biology to start a confidential conversation about your own risk. Having a tough time with this one? You might even rehearse in the mirror or in your head and say, "I have a family history of addiction to X substance."

CHAPTER TWO

The Accidental Discovery of an Addiction Predictor

Tell me about your childhood, and I'll tell you about your addiction risk

Vincent Felitti was starting to get hot under the collar—and it wasn't because it was one of those classic, hot Atlanta days. Felitti, a clinical professor of medicine at the University of California and the founder of the Department of Preventive Medicine at Kaiser Permanente San Diego, was wrapping up the final slide of an hour-long presentation to a gathering of his peers in the North American Association for the Study of Obesity. It was 1990 and the annual conference was his chance to show the culmination of an incredible year of research at his obesity clinic in California.

Nestled on the sixth floor of a palm-tree-lined street in San Diego, Felitti's clinic had achieved success helping clients lose hundreds of pounds using a new supplemented fasting technique. But Felitti's presentation wasn't focused on the before-and-after pictures and slimdown stories everyone loves to hear. Instead, he talked about the clients who had lost weight, left his program, and regained the weight they'd lost. One client had gone from 408 pounds to 132 pounds in less than a year only to start putting the weight back on as fast as she dropped it. Felitti went from reveling in his success, thinking, "We're going to be a world-famous clinic!" to shrinking from the disappointment and lamenting, "What the hell is going on here?"

Felitti was determined to figure out why solving the problem of obesity didn't, well, solve the problem of obesity for his clients. Why was the weight coming back? He decided to individually interview people who left the program and gained weight back again. Several weeks into his meetings, he asked a routine question that had a shocking answer. When Felitti asked a nurse's aide when she first started gaining weight, she revealed that it was at the age of eleven—when her grandfather began having vaginal intercourse with her.

What you have to remember in this story is that it takes place decades ago, when incest and sexual assault were rarely talked about. They were literally unspeakable issues that polite people didn't bring up. In his decades as a doctor, Felitti had only had one other case of incest—so he thought. So, when he heard another story of childhood sexual assault from a former client about a few weeks later—and another after that—he was stunned. One is by chance. Two is a coincidence. But three? That's a pattern. Could there be a link between sexual assault and weight gain?

He asked his colleagues for help with interviewing more patients who had left the program. They spoke with a total of 286 people and most of the time found the same shocking connection. So, in his groundbreaking presentation Felitti connected the previously invisible dots between the childhood trauma of sexual abuse and obesity. He also revealed that for many of these patients, treating their obesity didn't solve their problems. In fact, treating obesity *removed* the solution to their problems. Felitti

THE ACCIDENTAL DISCOVERY OF AN ADDICTION PREDICTOR

concluded that obesity helped them avoid unwanted attention, advances, and physical threats. Without it, they were vulnerable. As can often happen in Western medicine, he was treating the symptom (obesity), not the problem (unresolved trauma). Felitti didn't know what reaction he would get from his peers, but he certainly wasn't expecting disbelief, disinterest, or an ambush. During the presentation, one colleague actually stood up and claimed that Felitti was "naïve" and that doctors who were "more familiar" with the subject matter would recognize that the testimonies of his patients were lies to explain their "failed lives." Felitti was shocked that no one saw the psychological connection between sexual trauma and obesity. Until one person did.

Felitti later found himself at a speaker dinner that night with Dr. David Williamson, an epidemiologist from the Centers for Disease Control and Prevention, who suggested a solution to his problem convincing experts of the trauma connection: a larger sample size to show statistical significance. Maybe his group of a few hundred could be overlooked as chance. But interviewing several thousand people across the country? Similar results from thousands of respondents would mean the trauma connection was a genuine, giant red flag.

Together Felitti, Williamson, Dr. Robert Anda, another CDC associate, and other colleagues spent the next few years executing one of the largest investigations into childhood trauma and adult health. The 1995 Adverse Childhood Experiences (ACE) study included more than 17,000 people and looked at the impact of three types of abuse that happened to people before the age of eighteen: sexual, physical, and verbal. It also asked questions about other types of trauma, such as losing a parent. The survey was so controversial at the time that an Institutional Review

Board rejected earlier versions because of the sensitive nature of the questions. Even when the questionnaire was eventually approved, it required a rotating group of individuals working on the study to carry a cell phone twenty-four hours a day for three years to answer calls from people whose trauma was triggered by the questionnaire.

The researchers included multiple types of adverse childhood experiences in the study. Most likely to keep things simple, they defined a scoring system for the traumas that was based on whether you had a particular experience (like physical abuse) rather than how many times that negative experience happened. Originally, when they were still developing categories/questions, the highest score was eight. It became ten.

What they found astonished them.

The television fantasy of the happy American childhood was shattered. The link between childhood trauma and poor health outcomes was reinforced. Most of the people surveyed had at least one adverse childhood experience. Nearly a quarter (23.5 percent) had lived with someone with alcohol use disorder. A shocking 28.3 percent had experienced the physical abuse of someone slapping them, grabbing them, or hitting them so hard they were injured. And 23.3 percent experienced parental separation or divorce.

Through the analysis of the data, the researchers determined that the higher one's ACEs, the more at risk one is for serious health conditions like obesity, diabetes, and heart disease. The higher your score, the higher the number of sexual partners you were likely to have, which could increase your risk of sexually transmitted diseases and unintended pregnancies. People with six or more ACEs had a shorter life span—by decades. And, you probably saw this coming, the higher your score, the

THE ACCIDENTAL DISCOVERY OF AN ADDICTION PREDICTOR

higher your likelihood of developing a substance use disorder. As your ACEs increase, so does the chance that you develop an addiction to cigarettes, alcohol, or IV drugs. Their research found that a score of six meant you were 4,600 percent more likely to use IV drugs than someone with a score of zero. And, no, that is not a typo. You're *forty-six times* more likely. Since the 1990s, hundreds of studies have been anchored on this research, which initially looked at a score of six as the tipping point for diminished health outcomes as an adult. We've since learned through follow-up research that we need to look at a score as low as four as that tipping point.

Let's step back for just a minute. As a physician, when I review a research study, I look for the strengths of the study, but also its limitations. The strength of the original ACE study is that the sample set was large. A whopping 17,000 people! And like Williamson told Felitti, numbers that large do not lie. That said, while it was a very large sample set, it was not at all a diverse one. The 17,000 people who participated in the ACE study were mostly White, middle-class individuals with Kaiser Permanente health insurance. They looked a lot like the guys who were executing the study. Over time, researchers recognized this as a significant limitation and, in later versions, intentionally set out to ensure the population surveyed was representative of real-world populations. Through these subsequent studies, they found that certain groups are more likely to have experienced an adverse childhood event. They include people of color; lesbian, gay, bisexual, and transgender people; people who do not have a high school education; people who make less than $15,000 a year; and those who are unemployed or unable to work.

I want to be clear that Black people don't have more ACEs because they're Black and that LGBTQ people don't have more ACEs because they're LGBTQ. This data represents the result of systemic forces, like diminished access to resources and care, that culminate in ACEs. This problem is the result of racism, not race. It's the result of sexism, not sexual orientation. It's a result of classism, not class.

Nonetheless, in the '90s, despite the lack of diversity of the research, the outcome was clear. The higher your ACE score, the worse your physical and mental health and the higher your risk for substance use disorder. But why exactly was it happening? Why couldn't adults just shake off those bad experiences from their childhood? Why would ACEs have such a lasting impact?

The Science Behind ACEs

Most people have never heard of ACEs, are shocked by its accuracy, and aren't aware of its predictive power. There's some basic science behind why it's so eerily on point.

BIOLOGY. All of the childhood experiences we have train us both biologically and psychologically. We carry that training with us throughout life, the same way we carry the training we underwent to learn how to tie our shoes, ride a bike, and write our names without even thinking.

Maybe you're growing up in an environment where you don't feel safe because there's only one person there to protect you and they have to work double shifts. Or an apartment where you are constantly being yelled at or beaten for misbehaving—even when you're just being a normal kid. Or a house where someone is sneaking into your bed in the middle of the night and sexually assaulting you. That psychological

THE ACCIDENTAL DISCOVERY OF AN ADDICTION PREDICTOR

trauma has a direct impact on your biology. You're forming neurobiological pathways in reaction to your home life—and it has a lasting impact over the course of your adult life.

Another critical part of the equation is the fact that our brains aren't fixed for life. Many people are familiar with the idea that our brains are in a rapid period of growth and development from birth to adolescence. What fewer people realize is that that period of rapid development continues well into our late twenties. And what medical science has begun to uncover is that our brains have the capacity for change throughout our entire lives—even into older adulthood. This concept is neuroplasticity: the brain's ability to change its activity in response to environmental stimuli (like adverse childhood experiences) by reorganizing its structure, functions, and connections. If you're finding this hard to believe, consider that scientists can look at brain scans of people before and after weeks of meditation to show how mindfulness can change brain activity, increasing the size of the hippocampus (responsible for factual memory) and decreasing the volume of the amygdala (responsible for emotional memory like fear and anxiety).

That being said, our brains develop the most when we're children and adolescents. In a perfect world, you'd have a calm, stable environment where all your needs are being met as your brain is forming. But for many of us, our brain chemistry develops in a chaotic environment. We are small boats on a rocky ocean, and our brains feel and record every single wave because our family, our foundation, our survival is in jeopardy.

PSYCHOLOGY. As children, we develop our perspective on the world based on our life experiences. If you're growing up in an environment where you're abused, you might develop the perspective that "The world is a dangerous place" or "It doesn't matter what I do in life, I'll always get hurt" or "There's no way to get my needs met" or "I don't deserve to get ahead. This is what happens to people like me."

Now imagine carrying those thoughts with you into adulthood. If the world is dangerous, maybe you need ways to feel calm and safe and smoking marijuana helps with that. If being hurt is inevitable, then the dangers of IV drug use are just par for the course. Don't forget that, as I mentioned above, psychological trauma and perpetual fear can also impact your biology. Once your body gets used to the idea that you'll be on alert in fight-flight-freeze mode most of the time, it also leaves your blood pressure up, your muscles tense, and your blood sugar soaring. That can lead to a suppressed immune system, cardiovascular problems, and even cancer.

Something else is at play here, too. We're being set up in adulthood to re-create the patterns we were taught in childhood. Don't get me wrong. There are people who see a father with alcoholism and think, "I'll never be like that when I grow up." But many other people learn very early that alcohol is a way to calm fear in the brain and body that is in fight or flight mode most of the time. So, they unwittingly find themselves attracted to a partner who drinks heavily, and the cycle continues.

BEHAVIORAL. No matter how old you are, drugs can at least temporarily turn off the exhausting fight-flight-freeze response in your body. A glass of Cabernet or a Xanax can give you a break from feeling like you're running an emotional marathon every day. Stimulants, like Adderall, and amphetamines can turn up your adrenaline and make you feel like you're invincible and could run three marathons in a row if you had to.

THE ACCIDENTAL DISCOVERY OF AN ADDICTION PREDICTOR

At this point, if you're reading this book with a loved one in mind, you may have a bit of an enlightened grimace on your face as you connect the dots between what happened to them as a kid and what they're up against as an adult. If you're someone in recovery, I hope you have a sense of relief as you make those same connections. When I teach my patients about ACEs, I see the stigma and shame dissipate just a little bit. They take the first step on a journey from "This is all my fault" to "I'm not to blame for what happened to me in the past but I can take control of what happens to me in the future." In fact, it's your responsibility. From there, empowerment can begin.

What to Expect When You Take the Test

In this book, I address some of the heaviest topics out there in the lightest way possible with the hope of making difficult situations easier for you to understand and act on. For those of you who may be about to discover you have a high ACE score, I want to give you a bit of a compassionate trigger warning. I'm not saying that you definitely will have an uncomfortable reaction to the questions included in the ACE questionnaire. But some of the questions could cause you to remember traumatic experiences that you've tucked way back in the corner of your mind. They might cause you to feel intrusive or unexpected emotions like anger, sadness, or irritability. They might make you seriously rethink family dynamics that you believed to be normal or tried to forget about.

You may have the impulse to do something like I did when I took my first ACE questionnaire: Dive into a huge bowl of mac and cheese. I mean, they call it comfort food for a reason—neurobiologically, comfort food brings us a sense of safety. It's similar to the sense of safety many of Felitti's patients felt with their extra pounds. I've come to recognize an urge for mac and cheese as a cue that I'm under some sort of stress—even when I don't realize it. Not surprisingly, thinking through my childhood ACEs was stressful. Outside of cravings and impulses, you may feel physical sensations in your body as you go through the ACEs. Maybe you get a tightness in your chest, or your asthma starts acting up. Often, those are thoughts and emotions showing up physically in your body. It happens all the time, though many of us don't know to make the connection.

But doesn't it make sense that when you think about a surprising physical or emotional reaction you've had that there's important information about yourself on the other side of that? Don't forget that the ACE questions were emotionally liberating for many of the thousands of people who answered them. You may be about to read a question that could become your lightbulb moment. It might be that first step in a split staircase to understanding how the first eighteen years of your life impacted the next twenty. It could be just what you need to know to prevent it from negatively impacting the next twenty years of your life.

If you can feel your stress levels increasing as you read the ACE questions, or if you get an urge to skip a question (or eat mac and cheese), use that response as information and validate those thoughts and feelings. Something is happening that is worth exploring with a therapist or a faith leader in your community or a trusted friend. I'm going to urge you to send an email, pick up the phone and make an appointment, or go online for some counseling. Don't sweep those

THE ACCIDENTAL DISCOVERY OF AN ADDICTION PREDICTOR

feelings under the rug because now that they've been uncovered, I assure you they won't stay there. Find someone who can help you work through the heavy stuff, so you can come out lighter on the other end.

If, on the other hand, you are not stressed and discover that you have a low ACE score (three or lower), it's still important that you understand what's at play with other people and how they experience these traumatic experiences. That knowledge will enable you to help others, like the next generation in your family, keep their ACE score as low as yours is. Ready to dive in?

The ACE Questions

Give yourself one point for every yes answer and zero for every no.

While you were growing up, during your first eighteen years of life:

1. Did a parent or other adult in the household often or very often . . .
Swear at you, insult you, put you down, or humiliate you?
Act in a way that made you afraid that you might be physically hurt?

It's important to remember that anything that happens to our bodies in our physical environment also impacts our bodies physiologically. That's why when it's cold outside, you shiver. When you run up steps, you breathe harder. Now imagine that every time you get home from school and walk through the front door to your home, you're on edge or you occasionally shiver or twitch. And you don't stop until you leave the house the next day. Or that you're out of breath from the moment your dad gets home until he finally goes to bed. Is that your asthma or something else? Now remember that's every day for years. That's a long time for your heart, soul, and brain to be in a state of stress.

2. Did a parent or other adult in the household often or very often . . .
Push, grab, slap, or throw something at you?
Ever hit you so hard that you had marks or were injured?

Here, you can see the question escalates from verbal to physical abuse. And it's a similar impact. Verbal abuse frequently progresses to physical abuse, which can range from something as small as intentional pinching to life-threatening injuries.

3. Did an adult or person at least five years older than you ever . . .
Touch or fondle you or have you touch their body in a sexual way?
Attempt to or actually have oral, anal, or vaginal intercourse with you?

It's scary not knowing who might open the door in the middle of the night, climb into bed with you, and hurt you. This is what people normally think of when they think about child sexual abuse and that kind of experience is very traumatizing for a child. It's also scary for a child when someone encourages them to watch pornography or listen in on sexual acts. Or if someone watches them undress or use the bathroom. This non-touching form of child sexual abuse is a newer concept. Although it's not referenced in the question, if it's something you experienced, you would check "Yes" since we now know that non-touching child sexual abuse results in the same risk factors that touching does.

THE ACCIDENTAL DISCOVERY OF AN ADDICTION PREDICTOR

4. Did you often or very often feel that . . .
No one in your family loved you or thought you were important or special?
Your family didn't look out for each other, feel close to each other, or support each other?

As human beings, feeling nurtured is one of our most basic and primal needs. It's right up there with water, air, and food. Remember when we talked about how the dopamine pathway is committed to your survival? It's that part of you that tells your brain, "We need to be nurtured. We have to figure out a way to feel supported by someone. Never go without that feeling." So, when you don't receive that as a child, it feels like you don't have enough air to breathe. Or water to drink. This next question taps into basic needs going unmet as well.

5. Did you often or very often feel that . . .
You didn't have enough to eat, had to wear dirty clothes, and had no one to protect you?
Your parents were too drunk or high to take care of you or take you to the doctor if you needed it?

Again, we're tapping into needs we have as human beings, but this time it's the most basic things required for a sense of safety and to protect against addiction: food, clothing, healthcare.

6. Were your parents ever separated or divorced?

UN-ADDICTION

I'm not at all about to put any blame on parents who have decided to separate or get divorced. Many times, it is the absolute best decision they could possibly make for the sake of their children. But what I will tell you is that human beings are pack animals. And when one animal is removed from the pack, you see the impact on the rest of the pack. Losing immediate access to a member of the pack (through separation, divorce, military deployment, work opportunity) can be traumatic. Seeing a family member hurt or in danger can also be traumatic, which leads to the next question.

7. Was your mother or stepmother . . .
  Often or very often pushed, grabbed, slapped, or had something thrown at her?
  Sometimes, often, or very often kicked, bitten, hit with a fist, or hit with something hard?
  Ever repeatedly hit at least a few minutes or threatened with a gun or knife?

When people normally think of domestic abuse, they think of violence against women. But you should answer "yes" to this question if you witnessed any parental figure regardless of gender being pushed, grabbed, slapped, or any of the violence mentioned in this question.

8. Did you live with anyone who was a problem drinker or alcoholic or who used street drugs?

Risky substance use almost always contributes to unstable and unpredictable home environments. This can undermine a sense of psychological

THE ACCIDENTAL DISCOVERY OF AN ADDICTION PREDICTOR

safety, which is so important for predicting mental health and wellness in adulthood.

9. Was a household member depressed or mentally ill, or did a household member attempt suicide?

The fear and uncertainty associated with having a parent who is sick and unable to care for you can be carried into adulthood. Growing up in an environment like this could also lead to a fear of abandonment, fear of a parent dying, or fear of getting sick in the same way that your parent did.

10. Did a household member go to prison?

Imagine the rituals that a child gets used to from day to day of their father waking them up in the morning with a knock on their door, making scrambled eggs for breakfast, and then walking with them to school on his way to work. Now that ritual comes to an abrupt stop. There's no knock on the door at 6:30 a.m. The eggs aren't scrambled the way you like them. The walk is a lot faster because Mom has to be somewhere else.

That sense of loss can be crushing for a child. If the missing parent was the breadwinner, that's wildly destabilizing for the family as well. If others know about your situation, there can be an unbearable amount of shame. Maybe you have to deal with the fact that everyone in school knows your parent is locked up. And then when you get in trouble at school for grieving, people tell you you'll end up in jail just like your dad. And maybe you wanted to be like your dad.

UN-ADDICTION

Now that you're familiar with the questions in theory, let's talk about what they look like in my practice. I'm going to tell you a story about a man who had an ACE score of nine.

The idea of a family road trip probably makes most of us smile when we think back to our youth. But for my patient, Joseph, that's when all his troubles began. While his parents were busy navigating their way from Sacramento to Los Angeles, his adult male cousin was quietly molesting him in the rear seats of the station wagon. Joseph was only nine. That sexual assault was followed by others from a family friend. But when he told his parents, no one believed him. (If you're keeping track, that's two ACEs. One for sexual assault and the other for not feeling like your family looked out for you. In any relationship, safety matters first, and that was shattered for Joseph early on.)

While Joseph was in complete awe of his dad, and practically shadowed his father around the house, his father hated the attention, perhaps because he struggled so much to think that he was worthy of it. Providing for the family was hard. They moved to different, cheaper housing every other year and, at one point, had to stay with relatives for a few months while Joseph's father was incarcerated for possession of drugs that he was using to self-medicate his bipolar disorder. (A parent with mental illness and substance use disorder being incarcerated is three more ACEs, and Joseph is now up to five at the young age of twelve.) When Joseph's father was released from prison, the physical fights between Joseph's parents were nonstop and escalated to Joseph being verbally and physically abused as well. (That's six, seven, and eight.) When his father died of a sudden heart attack, fourteen-year-old Joseph witnessed his family fall apart. He was bounced from foster

THE ACCIDENTAL DISCOVERY OF AN ADDICTION PREDICTOR

home to foster home after his mother left to go to the grocery store and never came back. In the care of strangers who rarely treated him like their own child, Joseph often went to bed hungry and felt unsafe even after he aged out of the foster care system. (That's nine.)

After all that childhood trauma, it's not hard to see how Joseph was using cocaine by age sixteen. Followed by heroin a few years later, and amphetamines after that.

Fast-forward to twenty years later. When Joseph didn't show up for an appointment with me (he had never missed one in over a year), my team went out to look for him. He had been doing so well with his recovery. After a year of trying to get out of the trailer he shared with his cousin who was actively using substances, he, his partner, and their daughter were able to get their own house to move into. But then, under the weight of so many stressors and prolonged struggle, his illness relapsed. He overdosed in the bathroom while his daughter was in her room playing. Charged with child endangerment, he found himself in jail, like his father before him, wondering how he would piece his family back together.

I'm telling you this story not to tug on your heartstrings (okay, yes, to tug on your heartstrings), but also to ask you to step into the shoes of this human being and connect the dots between pivotal childhood experiences and adult outcomes. I want you to recognize that our childhoods so often turn into our adulthoods. I hope that you can understand that the unseen traumas people experience behind closed doors result in the traumatized person we see walking down the street. I want us all to find grace and compassion for the struggles that so many with addiction have survived, but not escaped.

Now what if I told you that Joseph's score isn't just nine. It's actually much higher—almost off the charts? Because while the ACE study was truly revolutionary at the time, no test is perfect. There were two deeply traumatic childhood stressors that were not included in the questionnaire.

The Missing ACEs

The original ACE questionnaire was laser focused on what happens inside of your household, so its original format pays little attention to formative events and outside circumstances that shape one's life. It goes without saying that a person's outside community and their peers can provide support and encourage health and happiness, but the world is a very big place. That outside community may have elements that are not as supportive and can destroy health and happiness as well. You may have grown up in a community where police violence against people who looked like you was an everyday occurrence or you were constantly followed around stores because clerks suspected you would steal something. In the original ACE study, racism and discrimination—two forces that can have tremendous impact on your life—weren't taken into consideration.

We're going to dive deeper into the physiology of this later in the book. But for now, what's important for you to understand is the impact these two forces have. Even if you can't relate to the experience of being mercilessly bullied on the playground because you keep your head covered in a religious observance or being traumatized by seeing someone get shot in a drive-by across the street from your corner store, all of us can relate to a time when we felt excluded or discriminated against.

THE ACCIDENTAL DISCOVERY OF AN ADDICTION PREDICTOR

Maybe it was by a group of kids who were more affluent than you or because you use a wheelchair. When you remember that the dopamine pathway craves nurturing, you can see how racism and an unsafe community cut that off. Now remember that your amygdala is deciding between fight or flight and all these dangers trigger anxiety. So, the message that your prefrontal cortex gets is "How can I reduce this pain?" And we all know at least one basic answer to that question.

Knowing what a significant impact peers and community play, the Philadelphia ACE Project took action. For the past ten years, they worked to expand the ACE questionnaire to accommodate for additional community-level stressors that particularly hit urban communities. Keeping those factors in mind, I'm leaning on their research and updating the ACE test for you to take here with five additional questions.

1. Overall, did you feel unsafe in the neighborhood(s) you grew up in?
Did you feel like people in the neighborhood(s) you grew up in failed to look out for each other?
Or did you see or hear someone being beaten up, stabbed, or shot?

2. Were you ever bullied by someone you didn't live with?
It could be a peer, a classmate, or an adult.

3. Did you often feel that there was no one in your life who helped you feel important or special?

4. Did you often feel that you were treated badly or unfairly because of your race, ethnicity, economic status, learning differences, or

other part of your identity?
This could also be your religion, gender, sexuality, or something else.

5. Were you ever in foster care?

Now that you've taken your score, the important thing to remember is that four or more ACEs is still the tipping point for those experiences having an adverse effect on your physical, mental, and even financial well-being. Ready for the part that might surprise you? My ACE score is five. That's right. FIVE. Seeing me from the outside, you might never guess that. And that's the point. Sixty-four percent of American adults have at least one ACE and 17 percent have four or more, like me. Here's how I get to my ACEs of five:

I remember what sounded like my dad throwing my mom up against a wall after an argument. I was just nine years old. I woke up the next day to a U-Haul truck in the driveway because my mom wanted to make sure a night like that never happened again. Eventually, after years of effort, they divorced. (That's two ACEs: violence and divorce.) My father was a Vietnam vet who was placed in the line of fire at just nineteen years old. He returned home with PTSD—before anyone knew what PTSD was. He was hypervigilant and easily triggered during the day; at night, I was told that he was prone to vivid dreams that could turn him violent. (Mental illness of a parent brings my ACE score to three.) Once, when I was five, someone sideswiped our car, hitting the passenger's-side door where I was sitting. My dad beat the guy up so badly, he ended up being the one sent to jail. (Incarceration of a parent takes me to four ACEs.)

THE ACCIDENTAL DISCOVERY OF AN ADDICTION PREDICTOR

My fifth ACE is tied to nights when the adults in my family were partying downstairs while us kids were upstairs listening to the swish of Hennessey being poured into a glass or the smell of marijuana wafting through the air. Sometimes I'd sneak downstairs to grab a snack or a piece of cake and see everyone having a great time. That was early in the evening. Then I'd fall asleep and be awakened by the sound of a drunken argument or a slamming front door. The real repercussions were the following day. In our house, we had a joke about "Calling Ralph." That's what my dad did most Saturday and Sunday mornings. He would get so high from drinking and smoking to self-medicate, the next day he was on his knees over the toilet bowl throwing up. (And that's how I arrive at five ACEs—someone in the household with alcoholism and/or using illicit drugs.) So, what enabled me to avoid the slew of statistics you've read that suggest I should be in a very different place in life? It's a little something called PCEs.

Uncovering an Antidote to ACEs: PCEs

If the ACE study is the most important test you've never heard of, it's about to get knocked out of that number one spot by PCEs. Pronounced "pieces," PCEs stands for Positive Childhood Experiences. The staggering data that has come out of the ACE study tells an important story—but it's only part of the story. Yes, there are people with a high ACE score who find themselves at greater risk for poor health, including substance use disorder, depression, cancer, and even poverty. But there are also people with a high ACE score, like me, who don't. It's not because I'm somehow superhuman or lucky. It goes right back to my childhood. If you can believe it, the same childhood that gave me a high ACE score gave me a high PCE score as well. As it turns out, even when the odds are stacked against you with adverse childhood experiences, there are seven positive childhood experiences (PCEs) that can help counteract that negative impact. Think of your ACEs like an overstuffed duffel bag that you have to lift up and carry through life. Your PCEs can function like wheels on the bottom of that duffel bag, decreasing the chance you sprain your back while carrying the load.

Researchers recently discovered that the positive interactions you had as a child, the strong bonds you created when you were young, and the valued support you were offered by others can lift you up—even while ACEs are trying to drag you down. Adults with PCE scores of six or higher were more than three times as likely to get the emotional support they need from their circle and 72 percent less likely to suffer depression and other mental health difficulties, according to a 2019 study published in *JAMA Pediatrics*. The lead author of that study, Christina Bethell, PhD, MBA, MPH, was instrumental in getting ACE and PCE questions added to the National Survey of Children's Health, an annual survey taken by tens of thousands of parents/caregivers that is funded and directed by the U.S. Department of Health and Human Services. It was a ten-year process, but she helped get this critical data included on the survey. Bethell is also a hopeful educator on and advocate for the power of PCEs. You've already learned that the presence of ACEs is detrimental to your health, but Bethell's research with her colleagues shows that the absence of PCEs can harm you as well.

THE ACCIDENTAL DISCOVERY OF AN ADDICTION PREDICTOR

Now I realize that the six out of seven score I referenced is a nearly perfect score and could be hard to obtain. So, it's important to note that a PCEs of three also makes a big difference, reducing your risk of mental health difficulties in adulthood by 50 percent. This reduced risk of mental health difficulties translates to a reduced risk of developing addiction.

While I encourage you, as well as all the parents I encounter, to intentionally strive to increase your children's PCE score, the effort shouldn't end when you hit eighteen. What I love about PCEs is that even if you didn't have these experiences as a child, it's never too late. Research shows you can still shore up your PCEs as an adult. And that only seems fair. While we can't control what happened to us as children, we have an opportunity to lessen the grip those experiences have on us as adults. Adding PCEs in adulthood will let you do just that. You'll want to aim for that tipping point of three PCEs to help move the needle toward your health and well-being. As I go through the seven PCEs, I'll explain how you can harness their protective qualities as an adult.

The PCE Questions

Give yourself a one if these scenarios happened to you often or very often. Give yourself a zero if it sometimes, rarely, or never was the case.

How often as a child did you . . .

1. Feel able to talk to your family about your feelings?

While we don't get to choose the family that we're born, adopted, or selected into, as adults we can decide who our chosen family or closest friends will be and who we will start a family with. The problem is many people unconsciously re-create the family they were born into. Becoming an adult and charting out on your own can be an opportunity to break the cycle, interrupt the pattern, and intentionally create something healthier and more supportive as an adult. Now, every single person who is part of your chosen family may not be able to be a sounding board for you. But you do need a few trusted allies that you feel able to talk to about your feelings and who will listen to you and provide support.

You can have the most amazing support system in the world, but if you're not able to communicate with them, it doesn't matter. Ultimately, your ability to articulate your feelings makes a huge impact. If you're not sure how fluent you are in the language of feelings, we'll tackle that shortly (see my suggestions on page 85). For now, just keep in mind that both access to support and ability to communicate with that support are key.

2. Feel your family stood by you during difficult times?

When you don't have to solve problems on your own, you're much more likely to find a positive solution. As a kid, that might be the parent who took your side when a teacher accused you of cheating or an uncle who showed up at the playground when you were being bullied. As an adult, that might be the partner who keeps you afloat after you get fired in a round of layoffs or the bestie who calls you every day when you're battling a bout of depression. I'm talking about your ride-or-die crew here. If no one comes to mind, it's time to work on finding them.

3. Enjoy participating in community traditions?
The key word here is "enjoy." When you're experiencing happiness, pleasure, or excitement by connecting with others, you won't be seeking out those feelings through substance use. When we think of a community, we tend to think about locations, but I'd like you to focus on the word "traditions." Perhaps this evokes memories of block parties in your neighborhood, Thanksgiving dinners, or going to see Fourth of July fireworks. Do you have similar traditions in your life today? As an adult, the traditions we choose can be critically important to our sense of connection, feeling supported and empowered. Think: Friendsgiving, an annual Gay Pride parade in your city, going on Bible school vacations, attending Alcoholics Anonymous or Narcotics Anonymous meetings, or an annual getaway with your closest friends.

4. Feel a sense of belonging in high school?
This question is all about the protection of connection, whether you played the trumpet and bonded with the other kids in your school band or you were understudy to Othello and felt a sense of belonging with the kids in drama club. For most of you reading this, high school is probably in your rearview mirror. But the need for belonging is very much in the driver's seat with you now. High school is just one pack. And it's in the past. Find your new packs now. They could be a work circle, a professional organization, the parents of your kid's friends,

diehard Atlanta Braves fans, or even people who love reading romance novels just like you. Belonging means that you can be who you are—unapologetically—with that circle.

5. Feel supported by friends?

Having strong friendships is a predictor of your wellness, with some studies showing that friendship is even more important than family in determining your happiness and health. If you haven't found your circle at this point, it can be really challenging to make friends later in life. But it's worth the effort. If you do have your solid circle, first make sure that it stays that way. The support you offer to others will be returned to you in-kind. Consider the love languages of your closest friends and lean into that when you offer support. Even though the classic book, *The 5 Love Languages: The Secret to Love That Lasts*, focuses on romantic relationships, it helps to consider which of the five languages speaks to your friends. Maybe they value gifts more than words of affirmation. Or they need quality time taking a yoga class with you more than they need you to put in the work helping them find a new therapist. The fifth language, physical touch, could be hugs, rubbing their back, or braiding their hair. Knowing how someone wants to be loved is just the first step. The next is knowing who you want to receive support and love from. You need to know who your go-to friends are for specific problems before the problem arises. The friend you can call and sob on the phone to for an hour when your dog dies might not be the same person who will drive over to your house and pack up all your clothes when you're breaking up with your boyfriend. Figure out your friends' strong suits and lean into them.

THE ACCIDENTAL DISCOVERY OF AN ADDICTION PREDICTOR

6. Have at least two non-parent adults who took genuine interest in you?

Once again, here are people who can pull you out of a difficult situation that could have led you down an unfavorable path. As a child, that might look like a teacher who encouraged you to study biology or a track coach who helped you increase your speed and enabled you to get a college scholarship. These people still show up in our lives as adults. They're the mentor at work who helps you get a promotion or the sponsor who helps you avoid taking a drink on a rough day. They're also people we pay to help us. That's right, even when you're paying for a service, people can take a genuine, vested interest in you. I do it with my patients all the time. Your therapist, your personal trainer, that career coach you hired? They're all rooting for you.

7. Feel safe and protected by an adult in your home?

Whether you're a child or an adult, if you're in a space that isn't physically or psychologically safe, the risk that you'll turn to other methods of escape (like substance use) is real. You'll know you're in a psychologically unsafe relationship if you worry about being ridiculed, insulted, or physically harmed by someone in your home. And you'll know if you've learned to create a psychologically unsafe space if you're doing those things to people in your home. While I know it can be easier said than done, it is extremely important that we choose partners who are nourishing and supportive—someone who creates a sense of safety for us.

4 Places to Find Real Friends as an Adult

There's nothing easy about making friends later in life. Everyone seems to be settled in their circle, but it is possible to create new connections. Here are the best suggestions I've found:

Look for People at Turning Points. Maybe they've just moved to the neighborhood or they're new to your church. Whether you're bringing them a welcome basket or asking them out for a cup of coffee after the sermon, take advantage of their desire to connect with new people.

Do Something New. On a Regular Basis. One patient of mine decided that twice a month on Saturdays, she'd go to a social event through Meetup. It took four outings (one hike, an art exhibit, a museum tour, and, finally, a musical performance) for her to find not one, but several people she clicked with. So, keep finding places to meet people in person and create real connections.

Consider Untapped Circles. Have you thought about seeking out friendships at your job? Could you connect with the teachers or other parents at your kid's school? Could you make a new friend through your AA or NA group? Sometimes the most obvious answers are right in front of us.

Ask Your Friends for Help. You'd call a friend and ask them to make an introduction if you were searching for a job or seeking a mentor. Why not ask them to connect you with other people they think you will click with?

THE ACCIDENTAL DISCOVERY OF AN ADDICTION PREDICTOR

Mind-Changing Conversation #2:
Speak Your Feelings and Support Your Friends

When you're feeling angry, scared, sad, or even joyful, do you reach for a glass of wine? Or smoke a cigarette? Or bust out the edibles? As you might have guessed, one of the biggest ways that we bypass or mute our own emotions is by using substances. Being able to talk to family about your feelings and feeling supported by friends are two important PCEs we've discussed that you can also lean on in adulthood to protect yourself (and your loved ones) from an increased risk of a substance use disorder. Picking up the phone or meeting up with someone can take the place of picking up a bottle of Jack or doing a bump of cocaine. Even if you feel like you've got this covered and don't use substances, I'm going to challenge you to take your skills expressing yourself to the next level with some tools I'm about to share. I want everyone reading this to be fluent in expressing their feelings. Let's start with a little exercise. I promise, it'll teach you something about yourself.

First, let me give you some background. Your brain and your body automatically react to stimuli in the following order: first, physical sensations; then emotions; and finally, thoughts. But as we become aware of our reactions, often we recognize our thoughts first, emotions second, and then physical sensations last. To illustrate this, I'm going to tell you a story and I want you to pay attention to what thoughts, emotions, and physical sensations you feel in your body as you hear the details. This will tell you a fair amount about how good you are at recognizing your feelings—and you have to recognize them first if you want to be able to express them later.

A young woman was meeting with her nurse care navigator during a routine check-in to see how she was progressing with her recovery from opioid addiction. A few minutes into the visit, they heard a thump. She hopped up, leaving the nurse in the kitchen, and ran into the bedroom. Seconds later, from the other room, she frantically yelled, "Oh my God! My boyfriend just overdosed!"

The nurse was able to calmly walk her through remembering where she had put the Narcan spray (an opioid overdose reversal medication which we prescribe for all our patients). Then he administered the drug, which blocks the effect of opioids and restores breathing, to her boyfriend. Within seconds, the woman's boyfriend took a gasp of air again.

When I tell you this story, what emotions are coming up for you? Take a moment to look away from this book and take stock of what your reaction is before you read further. You might be thinking, "I can't believe that happened!" Or "What a horrible situation." Maybe you're curious about the logistics: "I wonder what Narcan looks like?" or "I wonder if her boyfriend was on the floor?" You might be imagining how our patient felt: "I bet she was terrified!" or "I imagine she was shaking like a leaf."

If you found that you came up with a series of thoughts, take a moment to examine how you *felt*. If you had trouble tapping into the emotions that this story brought up for you, this may be a clue that you have a hard time tapping into your own emotions in general. What recognizing your emotions might have sounded like for some of you is: "I'm so angry this happened in the first place," "I was scared that person was going to die," or "I'm so relieved that he took that breath."

THE ACCIDENTAL DISCOVERY OF AN ADDICTION PREDICTOR

When You're Sharing Your Emotions with Someone Else

Think of a time when you experienced a strong emotion (like anger or joy) but didn't tell another person how you felt. It could be that you got extremely upset that your partner didn't help you with something or that in taking the ACE questionnaire you recalled a negative childhood experience. Or maybe you recall feeling happy about someone from your childhood who took an interest in you and was part of your PCEs. Or perhaps you thought of a favor a friend did for you that you haven't properly thanked them for yet. There's no statute of limitations on sharing and there's no time limit on talking about a feeling. You don't have to do it in the moment. In fact, delaying can work to your advantage. Here's how to work it into conversation with a supportive friend:

Pick the right time to talk.

It doesn't have to be as soon as you have the emotion. In fact, delaying your share could come in handy here because it gives you time to process your feelings. This is exactly why we tell people to count to ten or to do some deep breathing after something emotional happens, physiological grounding techniques to create the space to clear up your understanding of what you're feeling. So often, couples, for example, will avoid talking about serious topics when they're in a good mood, but that's often the best time to do it because you're not in that emotional state. You're calmer and better able to express yourself.

Give the person a heads-up and then dive in.

You might say something like: "Do you have a minute to talk?" or "You're going to laugh at this when I explain it, but I want to talk about something you said the other day." Or even "I've been working on understanding and expressing my feelings better and I'd like to try that right now with you."

Then you can delve into what you were feeling. You could say, "I was asked a question about my childhood yesterday and it brought back a lot of memories. I'm starting to feel depressed about some things that happened to me that I've forgotten about." Or "My initial reaction when you told me that you were too tired for sex the other night was anger, but when I thought about it, I realized that I'm scared that you're not as attracted to me as I am to you. And I know that's not true." Also, if the person doesn't have a moment to talk at that time, don't push the conversation forward. Wait until they are open to it.

Skip the apology.

Have you ever found yourself in the middle of telling an emotional story and then said, "I'm sorry. I won't burden you with this" or "I'm sorry I'm getting so emotional about this"? Not only do we censor ourselves when attempting to share emotions, we sometimes apologize for exposing and sharing our feelings in the first place. Now is your chance to stop saying sorry and start feeling supported.

Evaluate the exchange.

Did it go well? Then express your gratitude and offer to reciprocate. You could say, "Thank you so much. I'm so glad we had this conversation. It helps me to know that I can share my real self and my true feelings with you so deeply. And I want you to know that I'm here for you in the same way."

THE ACCIDENTAL DISCOVERY OF AN ADDICTION PREDICTOR

If it didn't go well, that's okay. If you feel upset—that's also okay. A coach my son had once said, "You're either winning or learning—and if you're learning you're winning." When it comes to building this muscle of self-expression, you're either winning or learning how to make that muscle even stronger. Not being able to share your emotions with *everyone* is a lesson we all learn. Not being able to share your emotions with *anyone* is a losing situation. In this scenario, the problem isn't that you shared your emotions, it's that this person wasn't able to receive that share. This moment is just insight that maybe for now, your mother, brother, partner, or friend isn't the right person to talk about your emotions with.

When Someone Else Is Sharing Their Emotions with You

If you're on the receiving end of a "Can I talk to you for a moment?" the goal is to be as fully present and compassionate with the other person as possible while they express their emotions. Maintain eye contact with them so they know you have their full attention, or consider placing a hand on their shoulder or knee if you know physical touch is one of their love languages. We're not taught to have engaged conversations like this. In fact, all too often, we're socialized into doing the opposite. So, I'm going to offer some suggestions of phrases you can also say to create a positive experience for your friend or partner.

Give them space to open up.

Accept the invitation to talk but take some pressure off of yourself. You could say something like, "I don't know that I have the perfect words to say right now, but I'm listening." That gives the other person permission to open up and lets you feel less like you're scrambling for something Oprah would say in return.

Validate that what they're going through is difficult.

It can be hard to sit in sadness and grief. As a result, instead of sitting in the difficult emotions someone brings up, we often try to change the conversation. If a friend shares that she just lost her job, you might accidentally say, "It's a great market, you'll find another one." If a relative tells you that he is struggling with a substance use disorder, you might say, "You can beat this! God doesn't give us more than we can bear." Despite good intentions, deflecting can be experienced as dismissive and invalidating. Instead, acknowledge what they're going through. That may sound something like, "This must be so hard for you" or "I can't even begin to imagine what you're dealing with."

Don't hide in humor.

Do you crack jokes when you feel the people around you are getting too emotional? Even if it's while watching a movie together, you feel like whispering, "What is this, a funeral? Let's cheer up!" You might say things like this in an effort to bypass your feelings of fear and cling to more positive sensations. If the temptation comes up to make a joke, take a moment to pause and identify what's making you uncomfortable in that moment. Is it that you're scared of saying the wrong thing? Do you pity people when they have emotional breakdowns? Are you terrified of being responsible for someone's emotional well-being? What is the emotion you're hiding from?

THE ACCIDENTAL DISCOVERY OF AN ADDICTION PREDICTOR

Embrace silence when it comes.

What would be your reaction if someone shared that their child died from a drug overdose? Sometimes when an unfortunate event happens to us or someone else, we feel the need to fill the silent weight of that event with words. If we keep talking—"Oh my goodness, I had no idea, if there's anything I can do to help please don't hesitate"—we can distract ourselves from our experience and the impact it's having. But what if we sat in that silence and explored our feelings? Instead, consider sharing one short sentence of comfort and then holding silence with them. Try something like, "I'm so sorry this happened to you and your family."

Let the tears flow.

We think that offering someone a tissue is the polite thing to do, but in reality, it actually is sending a message to that person to, well, shut up and stop crying. Not so sincere, when you think about it that way. "Clean yourself up and let's move on!" As an intentional strategy to let myself feel, I try to always let tears fall down my face for at least a few minutes before grabbing a tissue. I'd love for you to try it. When someone's opening up to you, keep that Kleenex to yourself and just hold their hand.

Un-Addicted: Your Inherited Psychological Risk

We just covered another key factor for addiction risk that you have no control over: your childhood mental health. This chapter may have brought back a lot of difficult memories, so let's take a deep breath, refocus, and recap what we can do about any damage that was done in your childhood.

Key Takeaways

> **Your risk of addiction is linked to your childhood experiences: ACEs and PCEs.**
> Your adverse childhood experiences (ACEs) and your positive childhood experience (PCEs) have a direct, scientific correlation to your health and wellness as an adult.

> **PCEs are an antidote to ACEs.**
> PCEs can mitigate the damage that ACEs have caused. While PCEs are not the opposite of ACEs and don't carry the exact same weight, they can significantly increase your resilience.

> **There's a way to increase your PCE score after childhood.**
> Positive *adult* experiences can function in the same way that positive childhood experiences do. Aim for a score of three or higher no matter what your age or the age of your loved one.

Your Homework

> **Partner up to take the ACE test.**
> Take the ACE test with a relative or loved one and share your answers. Not only can this help you remember incidents you may have forgotten, but it will also provide built-in support if you find it tough to complete the test.

> **Pay close attention to test question triggers.**
> If one of the questions brings back a memory that you've hidden away, talk to someone in your support system, such as a therapist, a religious leader, or a trusted friend.

> **Rig the odds in your favor for a higher score.**
> Pick one thing you can do every week to increase your PCE score. Journal about why that action is important to you and the impact it could have on your health.

> **Get fluent in speaking about your emotions.**
> It's never too late to have a safe space conversation with a trusted friend. Exercising your ability to do this can strengthen your ties to those around you.

> **Land on someone else's PCEs list.**
> Express a genuine interest in a child who may be missing supportive parental figures. Start a community tradition in your family or on your block.

CHAPTER THREE
A Garden of Eden for Rats
Why environment matters when it comes to substance use

"This is crazy," Professor Bruce K. Alexander frantically ran around telling anyone who would listen at Simon Fraser University in British Columbia, Canada. The year was 1982. The grant money he had been given by the university to study morphine use was being cut just as things were getting not just interesting but controversial. Without any outside funding, Alexander's research experiments would have to come to an end. "You can't do this!" he shot back at the administration. Unfortunately, as anyone who has worked in academia knows, he was wrong. The university administration pulled its funding, essentially sending a wrecking ball into one of Alexander's greatest achievements: a Garden of Eden he'd created for white rats that he nicknamed Rat Park.

No one knows exactly why funding got pulled. But it's not a stretch at all to say that the theories Alexander was investigating about what increases your risk of drug use were controversial at the time. This was the '80s, when the crack cocaine epidemic was approaching its height; the fried egg "This is your brain on drugs" commercial was running on repeat; and Nancy Reagan was perpetually telling people to simply "Just say no" to drugs.

A GARDEN OF EDEN FOR RATS

When he arrived at Simon Fraser University, more than a decade before Rat Park got torn down, Alexander had no intention to study addiction. He was focused on experimental psychology, a branch of the field dedicated to learning, memory, and cognition. But as the youngest assistant professor on campus, he drew that proverbial short straw and was assigned to teach an introductory course that no one else wanted: Social Issues. And you know what one of the biggest social issues of the day was? Heroin use. Back then, psychologists relied on flawed studies showing that heroin was irresistible once you got a hit. You're hooked and that's it. Those studies housed rats in something called a Skinner box, basically a metal enclosure three times their size with a little lever inside. The rats could press the lever and get a hit of morphine (which when processed for street sale becomes the opioid drug heroin) delivered through a small tube placed into their jugular that sent the drug directly to their brain. Rats would press that little lever over and over and over again. And there was the scientific proof that drugs were irresistible once you got a hit. Or were they? Today, we know that about 23 percent of people who use heroin develop an opioid addiction. The question many automatically ask is: What is it about the 23 percent that makes them so vulnerable to addiction but the remainder can experiment without any long-term consequences? But what if we shouldn't be asking questions about the person? What if we should be asking questions about the place where they live?

Even though psychologists were taught to think Skinner boxes were the proof, Alexander considered they were the problem. When he looked at the Skinner box, he didn't see a simple metal enclosure. He saw a prison cell. Solitary confinement. I mean, if you were trapped in a tiny box with nothing to do but drink water, eat food, or get a hit of morphine, what would you do?

After a few years of frustration with the old model of addiction, Alexander decided to experiment with something new. And that "something new" was Rat Park. In contrast to a tiny Skinner box, he created an 8.8-square-meter Garden of Eden for rats the size of his garage. Like a Skinner box, it had four walls. But those walls were plywood and painted with green trees meant to mimic the British Columbia Forest landscape. Rat Park was open air—it had no ceiling like a Skinner box so you could move in three directions. The floor was lined with cedar shavings to pile up, empty canisters to hide in, small boxes for nesting, and wire frame wheels to run on for exercise. And most important, there were other male and female rats to socialize with, fight with, mate with, and play with. Hearing the description of Rat Park, take a moment to think about that tiny box with the rat in isolation. Like humans, rats seek social interaction and connection. Robbing them (and us) of that can be devastating. Now think about the rats scurrying around with their friends, running on wheels and snuggling with each other. Seems obvious that the rats in Rat Park would use less heroin, right? But at the time, Alexander's results were shocking.

Alexander ran a series of experiments in which Skinner box and Rat Park rats were both offered a device for consuming morphine in their habitats. The morphine consumption of the rats in Rat Park was always a fraction of what the rats in the Skinner box consumed. That data held true even when he transferred a rat who had been consuming large quantities of morphine in isolation from a Skinner box into Rat Park. In one experiment, the isolated rats consumed up to sixteen times as much

A GARDEN OF EDEN FOR RATS

morphine as the rats in Rat Park. Perhaps addiction wasn't just about having access to a drug that then hooks you and you're done. Perhaps, Alexander showed, it was much more complicated than that. Perhaps addiction was a social and environmental problem.

Some experts have refuted Alexander's study, but others have replicated the results in ways I don't think anyone reading this book will find surprising. In a 2018 National Institute on Drug Abuse (NIDA) study (and yes, health officials should change the "A" from "Abuse" to "Addiction"), rats were given the option of pressing one lever for an infusion of heroin or methamphetamine or they could press another lever that opened a door so they could interact with another rat. Almost 100 percent of the time, the rats opened the door. In another study published in 2021 in *Frontiers in Behavioral Neuroscience*, some rats were placed alone in a chamber where pressing a lever administered cocaine and opened a door to another rat. Others were put in a chamber where pressing the lever administered cocaine but opened a door to something much less alluring on the other side: a black and white sock. The rats whose doors opened to a peer pressed the cocaine lever up to three times as much as the rats whose doors opened to a plain, old sock. So much for door #2. Are you noticing a social trend here? In my field we say that addiction is the epitome of disconnection and connection is the opposite of addiction. Those rats craved connection more than they craved drugs.

The Myths of Rat Park

It's no coincidence that rats are chosen for so many experiments. Over the decades, rats and mice have formed the foundation of much of our biological and genetic research that gets translated into human biology. We know that when a rat does X, that's the equivalent of a human doing Y. We call this translational research. At its core, the Rat Park experiment makes us aware that as social beings we are deeply impacted by our environments. That just like your DNA and your childhood experiences, the physical environment that you are in has a significant impact on the likelihood of you using drugs. Even if you've never thought of it that explicitly, you probably have experienced it. When you thought of that rat in the Skinner box, did you think of yourself during the pandemic? Because the parallel is clear. It's just that instead of having the limited choice of morphine or no morphine, we were presented with different limited choices in our Skinner boxes or homes. If you lived alone and had a stay-at-home order during the COVID pandemic with nothing else to do besides hop on Zoom calls with all your friends or sit by yourself, what did you choose? You probably pressed the "Start Meeting with Video" button. Over and over and over again. You might've even gotten "Zoom fatigue" but kept going back to the screen. At the end of 2020, Zoom reported sales were up a whopping 367 percent compared to the previous year.

If you lived with a partner and were stuck at home, is there anything you two were doing a lot more of? Because at the beginning of the pandemic, one study showed that 81 percent of people in relationships were having as much or more sex than before—of course an increase was more likely if you were in a positive relationship—and 20 percent reported trying something new in bed. That "something new" included everything from a sexual position to using marijuana or alcohol before sex. And those numbers continued to rise in 2021.

And I'm sure you saw this coming: in 2020, 13 percent of Americans said that they started or increased substance use to cope with the stress of the pandemic. When you think about yourself sitting around with nothing to do, you can probably imagine taking a drink or an edible to pass the time or disrupt that "is this how it ends?" stress loop in your brain. Perhaps that's part of the reason that liquor stores were considered an "essential business" during the pandemic. Simply put, when we were cut off from the unlimited options of the outside world (our Rat Park), we leaned into whatever or whomever was in our homes (our Skinner boxes).

If Rat Park was only groundbreaking for what it brought to light about socialization and environment, that would be enough. But there are some other revelations that I think Alexander's experiment shows us as well. Myths that will undoubtedly contradict what you have always thought about addiction. Let's keep our minds open like Alexander as I use Rat Park as a springboard for other surprising facts about addiction.

Myth #1: People who use substances don't care about themselves or their lives.

I know the types of things that people think to themselves when they see someone they love struggling with addiction. "Don't you get embarrassed walking around looking this way in public?" "Don't you want to hold down a job and be a part of society?" "Don't you care about yourself enough to take a shower?" The Rat Park crew—and the rats moved from Skinner boxes into Rat Park—imply that, yes, your loved ones do. Those rats scurried around mating, running on wire-frame wheels, and nesting even while they were using morphine in that Garden of Eden. But the Skinner box doesn't make that possible. It's hard to turn your back on the morphine drip when there isn't much else to do in your cage. And that cage can look different for everyone. It could be living in an impoverished neighborhood that has cheap, easy access to drugs on every other corner. Or growing up in an abusive home where there are plenty of prescription pills in the medicine cabinet. Or struggling with a mental or physical condition and having a doctor write addictive prescriptions without keeping a closer eye on you. People who use substances do care about themselves and their lives. But they might not have the environmental and social support to do so. Their own personal Skinner box may make it difficult to "choose" themselves over the drug.

By the way, I'm not just guessing at how these rats might feel if they were human. We have the data from talking to people who have a substance use disorder. In a first-of-its-kind national study, Community Catalyst partnered with the American Society of Addiction Medicine and Faces & Voices of Recovery (FAVOR) to learn from more than 900 people who have an addiction what mattered most to them in treatment and recovery. As doctors and professionals, we have ways of measuring how effective treatment is. But until now, it's never been reported what mattered from the perspective of people who use drugs. At the top of their list, as published in their "Peers Speak Out" report, was staying alive. So, yes, your loved ones do want to be here. Second was improving their quality of life and sixth was meeting their basic needs. So, yes, being a part of society and taking that shower? Both are important to them.

I want to share one more recovery factor that matters to people with substance use disorder. The fourth most important goal was improving their mental health. Most people think that when you have an addiction, it's one wild ride. Just party after party. But the truth is, people with active addiction are struggling. They might be depressed, anxious, having a tough time dealing with a life trauma. Their self-confidence and self-esteem have been stolen from them. And they want it back.

Their loved ones want something back, too. They behave as if they are frustrated, angry, and exhausted by people who have an addiction. But in reality, they are frustrated, angry, and exhausted by the fact that addiction is stealing our people from us. It's a thief in the night that we keep losing our loved ones to despite our outpourings of love, our own hypervigilance, million-dollar national campaigns, nonprofit organizational movements, and more. When I work with families, my primary goal is to help them focus their anger where it really belongs, which is on the addiction.

Myth #2: You have to hit "rock bottom" to change your substance use behaviors.

When people talk about hitting rock bottom, they usually mean a situation where all your basic needs (money for or access to shelter, food, water, nurturing) have been taken away. They tend to think of something they've seen in a movie or while driving by an underpass where someone is facing homelessness and hunger. But that's not a real rock bottom. Some Skinner box rats forgo food and water (technically hitting rock bottom) but still reach for the morphine drip. They die of starvation (their real rock bottom). The myth is, we think we know what someone's rock bottom is. The fact is that we have no idea. So much of what we might conceive as someone's rock bottom is not as bad as things can get. There's always farther to fall. I can tell you that death is the true rock bottom.

I remember a patient of mine whose youngest son was struggling with an addiction to opioids. His use caused him to lose his job and she had allowed him to live with her for several months, always believing that he would "pull himself together" tomorrow or the next day. Seeing that nothing was changing, her older son encouraged her to offer his sibling an ultimatum: go into rehab or get out of the house. No one in their family had ever been homeless, so they were sure that a night or two of hitting rock bottom on the streets would help him "snap out" of his addiction if he didn't choose rehab. Unfortunately, the young man refused rehab and started living on the streets, where he was violently assaulted and ended up in the emergency room minutes from death. Because the assault had been part of a brawl, he was arrested and taken to jail, where he got drug rehabilitation treatment that ultimately saved his life.

The point of this story isn't that you have to let your loved ones live in your home while they're struggling with an active addiction. In fact, it's important to avoid enabling life-threatening behaviors. The point here is for you to remember that you have no idea what someone's rock bottom will be—and that you should never wait for it or push them toward it. If a friend was diagnosed with stage 1 cancer and was terrified to get treatment, would you wait for them to hit rock bottom at stage 4?

Myth #3: It's impossible to use drugs without getting addicted.

As the Rat Park study shows us, it's much easier to use drugs without getting addicted when your environment supports your dopamine requirements. Certainly, some of the rats used morphine without getting addicted. And you know what else? I'll go so far as to say that if everyone could use drugs without harm, they would. How do I know? Let's look at it from another angle. This is an oversimplification, but I love chocolate lava cake. I know it may not be your thing. Maybe that's BBQ potato chips, skydiving, buying cars, or getting tattoos. But for me, it's chocolate lava cake. (Thank goodness it's expensive and full of sugar because if it weren't I'd have it all the time.) Now, if all of a sudden chocolate lava cake tasted just as delicious as I know it is, but had zero sugar and I could get it for free, I'd eat all the chocolate lava cake I wanted, right? Because there would be no repercussions on my diabetes risk, my dental health, or my bank account. But I don't eat chocolate lava cake nonstop because I already have more dental fillings than I care to share with you and my dessert budget (or lack thereof) is most definitely an ongoing discussion between me and my husband.

Now let's up the stakes a bit to smoking. What if you asked a crowd of one hundred previous smokers: "If you could smoke a cigarette without getting addicted, would you do it?" They'd probably say, "Yes. I liked the way it made me feel. It wasn't the example I wanted to set for my kids, but if a couple times a year I could smoke and not go to two packs, I would." Now drop in alcohol. Now escalate it to heroin. I know I fast-tracked us from that cake to heroin pretty quickly, but the idea is still the same. If everybody could use drugs without experiencing the harms of drug use, almost everyone would use drugs—there would be no reason not to.

The problem is, everyone can't. Even though the vast majority of people use drugs (from cigarettes to cocaine), there are still harms. "I've been sober for fourteen years," one of my patients told herself during the pandemic. "I can take one drink in the middle of this thing, and it won't make a difference." But that one drink quickly led her right back to two bottles a day and all the associated life difficulties.

Want more proof that if you could use drugs recreationally, just like those rats in Rat Park, you would? You probably already do. You just don't call it recreational drug use. But when you smoke a cigarette only after sex or just at parties, that's recreational drug use. If you drink alcohol only when you're at a family gathering or on vacation, that's recreational drug use. In fact, 84 percent of people age eighteen and older have drunk alcohol at some point in their life. But only 11.3 percent of Americans meet the criteria for alcohol use disorder.

All the drugs I just mentioned have a longer timeline to potentially taking your life. There are others with detrimental aspects that start to appear much sooner: Opioids and methamphetamines, for example, hit so much harder that there is, understandably, greater fear around them. But there absolutely still exists a sliver of people who use meth and heroin and are not addicted to it. That sliver is much larger for people who can use marijuana recreationally, for example. But it exists. Half of all people who used an illicit drug in the past year were not diagnosed with a substance use disorder. What will probably also shock you is that not everyone who has a substance use disorder has the goal of total abstinence. The majority of people recover to controlled use, depending on the substance. Read that last sentence again. It's true.

Myth #4: Drug use is abnormal and always detrimental.

Drug use is normal and can be beneficial. Record scratch. Wait. What did I just tell you? Yes. Drug use is completely normal and there are actual benefits to using drugs. Rat Park shows us how the rats normalized drug use to be recreational and still functioned. But the benefits might not have been so clear. When Alexander talks about the Skinner box, he says that taking morphine inside of one might have been "compensation for dislocation." He suggests that "we have to have a society that is fit for sobriety" in order to set our loved ones up for success. So, when you think about the rats, consider that the benefit of drug use might have been making them feel better about the terrible cage they'd been put in. When you're in an environment that steals your sense of joy and purpose, or you're in a place that doesn't allow you to have fun, you create a dopamine deficiency in your brain. That deficiency can feel like a threat to survival that triggers the amygdala. And one solution is alcohol or drug use. All drugs will interrupt that cycle of deficiency for every single person.

But there are other benefits we rarely talk about because it's so tempting to see drug use as black and white. It's all bad, when in reality, it may be helping a single mom feel less tired so that she can work an extra shift and bring home more money to her family. It could be giving an awkward kid the calm he needs to socialize with his peers instead of letting anxiety get the best of him. Or perhaps it's helping your partner manage his anger, so he doesn't come home at the end of the day and spark a fight.

One patient of mine was a veteran of the war in Iraq. She came back to the states with PTSD that, like so many of her fellow veterans, was diagnosed but untreated professionally. Instead of medication, she turned to drinking gin and smoking marijuana to keep the flashbacks of IEDs taking the lives and limbs of the soldiers she fought alongside. Eventually she was spending her family's rent money on alcohol and weed, which led to drunken arguments with her husband that often escalated into her throwing punches. When she came to me for help, she set a goal for complete abstinence, so we knew we had to address the PTSD in some other way to get her relief. I prescribed an antidepressant (biological support) and we did talk therapy (psychological support) to help her heal from her violent experiences. She worked with veterans coming back from deployment, sharing her own experiences and encouraging them to get the support they needed upon return to ease the transition. Do you see what happened there? We changed her environment and social circle. We empowered her by having her volunteer and interact with others who understood her experience and could benefit from her journey. If we hadn't created that Magic Formula™ for her, there was a high risk her addiction could have relapsed in no time flat.

Drugs have pros until the drugs become the problem. But we can't simply take drugs away from people once drugs become the problem. My patients often say, "I thought if I just quit using, that would fix everything." That's not the case. We have to recognize that drug use initially had benefits and served a purpose of some sort. We need to

A GARDEN OF EDEN FOR RATS

replace drug use with something else so that people can get those benefits elsewhere: therapy, safe prescription medications, social support, community traditions, environmental shifts, life meaning and purpose. If we don't, we are begging their addiction to relapse to meet those unmet needs.

Like the rats in the Skinner box, humans have the power to create environmental conditions that pressure us toward regular drug use and drive addiction—especially if there's a biological disposition toward addiction. We also have the power to create environments where drug use is as recreational as the rats running on a wire-frame wheel. But we don't have to rely on animal studies entirely to see how environment impacts our health and risk of addiction. Let me tell you about your ZNA.

Your Zip Code Is More Influential than Your Genetic Code

Earlier I told you that 40 to 60 percent of your addiction risk is inherited, coming straight from your DNA. However, when it comes to your overall health and longevity, experts believe that your DNA plays a smaller role of about 30 percent. The remaining 70 percent has to do with the environment you grew up in. That includes everything from your economic class to your access to healthcare to whether the water in your neighborhood is safe to drink. Researchers call this your ZNA.

Experts created the term ZNA to represent your zip code at the time of your birth. Researchers often look at and refer to zip codes as being the geographic determinant of health as well. Turns out zip codes very accurately predict how our environment gets coded in us and the impact that can have on our health. If you're like me when I learned about ZNA, you're itching to google your own zip code for a glimpse into the future of your health. Pair that with a 23andMe kit along with ACE and PCE scores, and you'll have almost everything you need to know to understand your risk for developing addiction.

But here's the thing. We all inherently know that environment has a big impact on our health; it's just something zip code data helps us prove. Anyone who has ever thought of moving to a "better" neighborhood so their kids have access to a great education or more outdoor space to play in knows that environment matters. And they're right. Research shows that being raised in a neighborhood with high rates of poverty and unemployment (compared to an affluent neighborhood) can lower your chances of getting a high school diploma from 96 percent to as low as 76 percent. It's not hard to imagine the cascade of economic, social, and environmental limitations that follow.

My family and I have chosen to live in a nearly completely Black suburb of Atlanta, which means that the value of our home is lower (nearly 75 percent lower than the exact same home just eight miles up the road); our tax base is smaller, which results in less funding for our public schools; and my oldest son goes to a high school where the majority of students are eligible for free or reduced lunch. When the pandemic hit, the zip code divide hit us square in the pockets. If I were ordering food delivery for my family, every single option was pizza, wings, and burgers. I realized that we are essentially in a food desert (an area where access to healthy, affordable food is limited) unless you can afford to pay an extra fee for being out of the delivery zone—and

A GARDEN OF EDEN FOR RATS

by extra, I mean like $12.99 on an order that costs $20. That's basically a healthy food tax on a zip code of people who are already disadvantaged. Our privilege is being able to afford that fee. Most of my son's schoolmates are not so privileged. And we all know how important access to good food is: all humans need the building blocks of nutrition to fight disease, keep our brains sharp, regulate our hormones, give us energy, and so much more.

The difference that a few blocks can make is shockingly apparent when you look at one particular neighborhood in New York City. While you won't find an actual concrete wall spray-painted with graffiti art there, Manhattan did have a stretch of city blocks that used to be ominously nicknamed "The Berlin Wall." East Ninety-Sixth Street, between Fifth Avenue and the East River, was an invisible, but very apparent, dividing line between two regions in the mid-2000s. To the south, there were the more affluent and predominantly White neighborhoods of Carnegie Hill and the Upper East Side. To the north, as soon as you stepped past Ninety-Sixth Street, you'd find the more diverse and less prosperous neighborhoods of "El Barrio" or East Harlem. That invisible line, as recently as a little over a decade ago, marked a stark end to sightings of beautiful high-rises and posh eateries and a rapid uptick in the amount of rundown public housing and check cashing establishments you could count. Go a little farther back in time and you'd see a slew of White faces getting off the New York City subway at the Ninety-Sixth Street stop as the train shot farther north with the remaining Black and Brown passengers.

What you couldn't see, until researchers started crunching massive data sets, is that the Great Divide at Ninety-Sixth Street didn't only decide whether your local movie theater had plush recliner seats, or the mac and cheese at your corner store was made with Gruyère, or whether or not you could hail a yellow cab if you were in a rush. The invisible line wasn't just about economics. It was also about survival. It marked how long you could expect to live.

The United States Census Bureau has been collecting regional data for more than a hundred years. In the past few years, the City Health Dashboard (created by NYU Grossman School of Medicine's Department of Population Health and with support from the Robert Wood Johnson Foundation), along with other research organizations, such as the United States Small-Area Life Expectancy Estimates Project (USALEEP), looked at population information and death records according to census tracts. What the projects' analysis revealed to the public was that *where* you live at birth can dramatically impact how long you can expect *to live*. Living a few blocks in one direction could take up to *thirty years* off your life. This analysis led to other studies that investigated what aspects of a physical environment could contribute to those lost decades.

That Great Divide on East Ninety-Sixth Street marked a life expectancy difference of more than eighteen years. People residing south of it in the Carnegie Hill area had a life expectancy of 84.9 years. But those residing just three city blocks north of it, in East Harlem, had a life expectancy of 66.2 years. Disparities like this play out across the United States. In Atlanta's Bankhead neighborhood, life expectancy at birth is 63.6 years, but just three miles to the east, a section of the Old Fourth has one of 80.5 years and farther north, the posh Buckhead neighborhood residents can expect to live 80.9 years. In Chicago, the difference is the largest in the country, with a life expectancy gap of

A GARDEN OF EDEN FOR RATS

more than thirty years between the neighborhoods of Streeterville and Englewood, which are less than ten miles apart. Crazy, right?

What I want to make sure we focus on is not just the "what" of what's happening but also the "why." Why are people dying thirty years sooner? What are the root causes? In the East Harlem area, unemployment is at 16.8 percent—almost three times the rate of joblessness just three blocks south in the Carnegie Hill section. If you don't have a job, you may not have access to healthcare or money for healthy food. In that section of East Harlem, high school completion rates are at 69.4 percent compared to 99.5 percent in the Carnegie Hill neighborhood. Pretty hard to find a high-paying, safe job without a high school diploma. In the East Harlem area, lead exposure is higher and obesity levels are almost double while routine primary care checkups are lower.

Speaking of addiction specifically, another way we know that we inherently recognize the power of environment on our health is the classic mantra: people, *places,* and things. Twelve-step programs, like Alcoholics Anonymous, are abstinence- and faith-based recovery programs that take you through twelve steps (like admitting powerlessness over addiction and making amends) to support your recovery. They are also the source of the People, Places, and Things mantra that helps its members identify triggers for their substance use. One of the reasons that destination recovery centers have such a high rate of success while patients are on-site is that they remove environmental triggers, which can be the cause of up to 60 percent of the relapse risk for an addictive disorder. You're no longer a phone call away from your dealer or a block from the local liquor store or a car ride away from the friend you use with on the weekends or drowning under the cumulative daily stress of too little time and too little money. Instead, you're in a relaxing environment with a strong support system, medical support, and time and space for mindfulness. Why wouldn't recovery work under those circumstances? But when you come back to your "real life," a whole new level of coping skills and ongoing support is needed to keep your illness in remission. And this is where we often drop the ball, thinking thirty days away was the cure, rather than just the first step of an ongoing journey.

Even if you're not in recovery from an addictive disorder, geography can impact your use of substances. In that Carnegie Hill area, only 6.7 percent of residents report smoking. In East Harlem, 19.7 percent do. On top of that, just stepping two blocks north of the Carnegie Hill area leads to a more than 5 percent increase in self-reported binge drinking. Again, it's important to look at not just what's happening, but why it's happening. And one reason for that might be proximity and access. Living or going to school near a liquor store (roughly within 800 meters) increases a teenager's likelihood of drinking alcohol. Research has shown higher rates of pedestrian injuries and drunk driving accidents in neighborhoods with a greater density of liquor stores. One study looked at more than 1,600 zip codes in California to determine that the more liquor stores there were in a neighborhood the higher the number of childhood accidents, assaults, and child abuse injuries in that area. This certainly sounds like a complex interaction of environmental factors and ACEs to me. I imagine a type of vicious cycle. Parents trapped in the Skinner box of high-demand, low-wage jobs stopping by the local liquor store on the way home to ease the

A GARDEN OF EDEN FOR RATS

stress of the day. Some days, the stress is so high, they crack open the first beer in the parking lot, increasing the risk of a drunk driving accident and arrest. Kids left at home alone as their parents work hard to make ends meet; surrounded by liquor stores instead of playgrounds, they get into all sorts of interesting but risky things that lead to accidents and fights. An already stressed to the brink parent gets the call about an injury that they have neither time nor money to address, and the frustration boils over. What's meant to be discipline turns into abuse. Biologically predisposed, beaten down, and unable to talk about their feelings with their parents, the teenagers turn to alcohol—from the local liquor store—and the rest of the story continues to write itself.

The data looked similar when access to cigarettes and marijuana was analyzed. High levels of places to buy tobacco in a neighborhood resulted in high levels of kids smoking. An increase in the number of medical cannabis dispensaries in an area led to an increase in hospitalizations for cannabis use disorder in the following year. And why wouldn't it?

If every time you're on your way home from school after getting bullied, you pass by five liquor stores, you might stop in one to try to get a bottle of *anything* without the clerk IDing you. But what if you passed by five basketball courts instead? Or five after-school centers where other kids were learning to play chess? Or what if your parents had the time to pick you up and drive you home?

When Your Environment Actually Changes Your Biology

It's pretty easy to see anecdotally and hypothetically how where you live impacts your physical health. But I also want you to be aware of direct connections that have been found by scientific research. One study looked at brain scans of a small group of young teenagers who were exposed to community violence like hearing gunshots outside their window, seeing someone getting beat up at the park, or witnessing illegal drug use while they're on their way to the corner store. The study found that the teens' amygdalae (emotional memory such as fear and anxiety) and their hippocampi (factual memory) were smaller in volume compared to those of teens who said they saw less violence in their community. In other words, environmental stress created psychological stress that changed the biological development of the brain.

And get this: Not only do community violence and other types of traumas change your brain, they also impact your DNA. Research on the children of Holocaust survivors has shown that trauma can be passed down to children even after the event through their genes, which researchers refer to as epigenetics. These epigenetic changes don't change the DNA sequences in your body, but they can alter the expression of a gene. For example, turning it on or off, making you more susceptible to stress and depression or more likely to be resilient.

Another study I'll tell you about will make you wish we were back to experimenting on rats and not people. It's the 1994 Moving to Opportunity study. In Baltimore, Boston, Chicago, and Los Angeles, nearly 5,000 families in poor neighborhoods were randomly assigned to one of three groups. The first group got financial vouchers that they could only use to subsidize housing in a more affluent neighborhood. The second got vouchers they could use in any neighborhood. And the third received no vouchers. Pretty tough luck in the name of science. But I'll still tell you the outcome: the families that moved to more affluent areas had lower rates of obesity and diabetes than the families that moved from one high-poverty neighborhood to another (remember my food delivery anecdote earlier?). There's environment impacting biology once again. What grocery stores and restaurants do you pass by in your more affluent neighborhood? What happens to your stress levels when you're not hearing gunshots at night? Or when the nearest stress reliever is a basketball court or yoga studio rather than a liquor store? Biological. Psychological. Environmental. It's all connected. But for now, let's talk about how you can exert a similar amount of influence over the environment that's influencing you.

Mind-Changing Conversation #3: Are You a Flower ... or a Weed?

There are two images I like to show when I'm giving PowerPoint presentations to capture how we've been taught to ignore the impact of environmental influences on our health. Since you're not staring at a screen in the dark surrounded by doctors and healthcare professionals, you'll just have to imagine that I've clicked a pointer and pull up the first slide in your mind. The image is of a beautiful garden with a vibrant flower growing in it. That flower has deep green leaves, soft pink petals, and even a few thorns to protect it from harm. The next image is of a weed that has popped up through a crack in the sidewalk pavement. The colors aren't so vivid, the bloom of a flower isn't there, and our instinct is probably to figure out how to pull it out or spray it with something so it dies.

I show that image to remind people that we tend to think there's something better about that luscious plant. We believe that it's superior to the weed because we don't consider the environment that the plants were brought up in. That flower had all the advantages of perfect soil and unlimited sunlight. But the weed had to survive much harsher conditions and squeeze in between pavement stones just to get a little sun—only to be sprayed with vinegar or plucked out by a gardening glove. (And, yes, those are metaphors for addiction and gun violence.) Isn't there something more impressive about what the weed has achieved through perseverance compared to what the flower accomplished through ease? Those weeds are people who have had environmental risk factors stacked against them. They are survivors. Imagine how they could flourish and flower, if we could just get them into a lush garden with nourishing soil and unlimited sunlight.

Changing the way we think about those flowers and weeds is just the first step. Now let's change the way we talk about them. And to do that, I'm going to ask you to have some really tough conversations.

First, a Conversation with Yourself
Question #1: *What soil was I planted in? How did my environment impact me back then?*
When you think back to being a kid, what was your physical environment made up of? Do you now notice how many liquor stores were in

A GARDEN OF EDEN FOR RATS

the neighborhood you grew up in or how often you saw little baggies at the local playground? Do you remember being able to ride your bike anywhere carefree and only once or twice seeing someone drinking out of a paper bag on the street? Did everyone have their own bedroom? Did you have a front yard to play in? Or was space scarce, so it was at least two to a bed and the playground was a long walk away?

One of my colleagues is the CEO of a multimillion-dollar company who can regularly be found at conferences in a suit, tie, and shiny wingtip shoes. But he'll tell you, somewhat apologetically, that he likes dirt, loves being in nature, and often has to get away from the city to do it thanks to his small-town, farm-rich upbringing. The part that gets to me is how apologetic he is about it when research shows how good this is for you. We know how normal it is to be in nature. But even when our environment is good for us, we are sometimes taught to reject it.

Like my dirt-loving colleague, I'm a lover of the great outdoors. I grew up in a suburb of Indianapolis, and right behind our backyard was straight up woods and nature. My brother and I would spend hours wandering through the trees and bushes to a nearby creek, stopping along the way to notice strange plants, discover colorful bugs, and even take home some wild animals. A few times my brother actually brought home turtles and (wait for it) snakes from our adventures in the woods. And my parents let him keep them. We got to explore those woods and the streets of our neighborhood, which were lined with crab apple and mulberry trees we could pick from without any worries. It was a safe physical environment where we were never bothered by anyone—especially not the police. It was all fresh air, sunlight, nature, and expansiveness. We could just be.

Fast-forward to the soil I'm currently planted in, which is less like the one I grew up in. It's still suburban but there are no woods right behind my house. But when I get away for vacations, I almost always look for something expansive where I can climb to a mountain peak or lie on a beach, or head to the top of a high-rise and enjoy being in the sky. I look for places that feel like the middle of nowhere but are actually in the middle of somewhere. (I mean, I do like amenities.) And I wouldn't be surprised if it makes my blood pressure go down, helps my breathing get deeper, and strengthens my sense of calm.

You can't change your childhood, and so we would never set that as our goal. But you can learn from your childhood environment. Think about what helped you thrive and strive to re-create that in your current environment. That's exactly what I'm doing when I lean into expansiveness each time I get away from my everyday environment. Also give yourself time to think about negative risk factors that we may have overlooked in our childhood environment and consider their possible impact. Use those as clues about what you want to avoid re-creating in your current environment and what might be triggers you need to eliminate now.

Question #2: *What soil am I planted in now? How is my environment impacting me now?*

I'll tell you a secret about Rat Park. Even if you think you're one of the lucky ones and you're in your own Rat Park with plenty of sunlight, gyms, and comfy places to nest, there's a chance you're actually in the Skinner box. One way to tell is to imagine where you'd like to go for your next vacation. Did you immediately envision a staycation inside

A GARDEN OF EDEN FOR RATS

the four walls of your home where you could just kick back and relax? Yeah, I didn't think so. Chances are, you pictured an emotional and physical getaway—someplace where you could get a lot more time in the great outdoors whether you were on ski slopes or lying on a beach. You might've imagined someplace where you could soak up the sun and strike up a conversation with a stranger at a beachside bar in Maui. Or perhaps you saw yourself leaving a seafood buffet on your way to catch a show in Vegas. Maybe you enjoy an adrenaline rush and thought about going skydiving or bungee jumping. We use our vacations to break down the walls of that Skinner box and escape to Rat Park.

Now that your real Rat Park is front of mind and your everyday life Skinner box is coming into focus, take note. Are you living alone in a tiny studio, or in a project apartment packed with other people? Are you feeling isolated living in the suburbs and wishing you had more meetups with friends or could get away to go on hikes every weekend instead of having to work on the house? It's important for everyone to get a break from their Skinner box—even if it's in very small ways.

First, write down three things about your current physical environment that could drive your (or a loved one's) risk of substance use. Think about all the spaces you might inhabit (home office, living room, bedroom, bathroom, work office, lunch break at work; a friend, parent, or relative's home; your car or a vacation) and journal about potentially addictive behaviors that are tied to them.

For example, are you more likely to take a drink when you have a beautiful wine rack on your kitchen counter? Do you have a greater desire for smoke breaks standing outside the building at work compared to when you're at home because that's where everyone else does it? Is there a pretty good chance you'll do a line of cocaine when you're hidden away in your neighbor's finished basement that has no windows?

Now you want to use that information to make intentional decisions about your environment. One of my former patients who has an alcohol use disorder struggled with abstaining on her ride home from work. It wasn't the stress of the day that got to her, but the signs for the exit where she used to pull off to get discount bottles of alcohol at a liquor store. Five days a week, she was testing this willpower to keep driving instead of taking the exit and bringing home bottles of club soda and vodka. So, we made a plan to change her environment. She couldn't change where the liquor store was, but she could change her route home from work. We plotted a different route that didn't require her to pass by that triggering exit. And it worked.

Simple changes like that can work for you, too. That wine rack on the kitchen counter can get tucked away in a cupboard. The apartment that's too small for the number of people living inside can be escaped for an hour by taking a long walk in the park after dinner every night to reduce stress. For every environmental risk you jot down, try to also write down a change you can make to lessen that risk. How can you get yourself to a space where you feel fulfilled? Creating and having choices is a source of power and control.

It doesn't go without saying that you'll want to get rid of things inside your house that are tied to using. If you're going to stop smoking marijuana, that decorative bong on your shelf should find a new home at the top of the closet or the bottom of a garbage can.

A GARDEN OF EDEN FOR RATS

If small changes aren't enough and you're struggling with a substance use disorder, you may need to radically shift your environment. A rehabilitation center outside of your current environment can physically separate you from the people, places, and things that drive your addiction. You'll get a resilience boost and lengthen your psychological bandwidth by stepping outside of your Skinner box. Keep in mind that you need to have support in place back home after the (typical) thirty days because just like a five-day stay in the hospital doesn't cure diabetes, a thirty-day stay in rehab doesn't cure addiction. No matter what environment you're in, you'll need ongoing biological, psychological, and environmental support systems to help you achieve and maintain your recovery goals.

Second, a Conversation with Others in Your Life
Question #1: *What soil were you planted in as a kid? Were you a weed or a flower?*

You've already done this work on yourself, but now it's time to have the same conversation with the people that you share your home with. Share your own story so they can get an idea of how to analyze their own lives and the environments they grew up in. Then use that information to carry the conversation forward.

Question #2: *What soil are we planted in now? What are some things about our environment that make you wilt? What are some things that make you blossom?*

Not everyone's answers are going to be the same even though you're living in the exact same location. What might be stifling or feel toxic to you may feel thrilling or life-giving to someone else. So, it's important to hear all your cohabitants out. Then, take action. Even if you can't afford to move to a different neighborhood, you may be able to change your environment for an afternoon or a weekend. Plan a picnic or pack a book to read at a park or beach in a neighborhood that brings you calm or joy. Drive or take public transportation to a nature trail or go on a cheap boat ride. You can also try looking for organizations that might be putting together events for you or the young people in your life. Perhaps a local church is organizing a day trip for apple picking or a not-for-profit youth development organization is sending kids to camp for the summer. Once you start googling resources, you'll be surprised by what appears.

If you've got some cash that you can put toward an environmental shift, consider pooling resources with your neighbors. You can chip in together to rent a car and a hotel room to get out of town for the weekend. Be intentional about it and share with them what you've learned about how all these things impact your health and the health of your family—and invite them on your journey. You can say something like, "I'm not going to be around at the end of this month because I'm taking a day-trip out of town. I read about how much our neighborhood can impact stress and decrease health and I want to do something to balance that out. Want to come? I'd love the company."

Un-Addicted: Your Inherited Environmental Risk

At this point, you've been introduced to the three pillars of addiction risk that are riddled with misconceptions: biological, psychological, and environmental. No doubt you're beginning to look at your childhood home, your current living situation, and the neighborhoods of your friends and family a little differently. You've probably even googled the health statistics for your zip code.

Key Takeaways

》 **Your risk of addiction is linked to your environment.**
Just like the rats without a Ferris wheel, human beings can turn to substance use when they lack space to socialize, exercise to de-stress, and ways to entertain themselves. But even when you have those things you can still feel trapped. Notice the clear relationship between you or your loved ones feeling like you're in a Skinner box and a desire to use substances or engage in other addictive behaviors.

》 **Drug use is most often recreational.**
We're taught to think of substance use as a harmful act, but research shows millions of people use substances every year without incurring any harm. Maybe you found yourself clinging to the benevolence of your evening glass of Chardonnay a little tighter than you'd like to admit, imagining that someone else using illegal drugs has more of a problem than you do? This is one of the ways we convince

ourselves that "they" have a problem and "we" don't. It could be that neither of us has a problem. It could be we both do.

> **Drug use can be beneficial.**
We're taught to exclusively think of substance use as always having terrible drawbacks, but the reality is that there are benefits to using substances for many people. From being social lubricants to easing anxiety to helping us think more clearly, many Americans see the positives in drug use. The key for all of us—and especially those of us with an increased risk for substance use disorders—is to recognize when our substance use is turning into preaddiction or addiction. At that point, you need to figure out how to get the benefits of the substance from something less harmful.

Your Homework

> **Create a crisis coping list.**
Consider your strategies for dealing with work drama, family problems, or even the never-ending cycle of depressing news and make a list of the ones that turned out not to be so helpful. The goal is to minimize less helpful solutions (like bottomless nachos) and add more positive ones (think morning meditation) to your tool kit.

> **Shift a behavior to beat your environment.**
Create a list of seven ways (one for each day) in which you can change how you engage with your environment to decrease your risk of substance use. That might mean picking a different route home so that you don't pass by marijuana dispensaries or skipping a boozy brunch and going for

coffee and a walk in the park with a friend. It could mean never bringing beer home from the supermarket so it's not readily available in your fridge at 2:00 a.m. or working through the smoke breaks your coworkers take at your job.

》 **Uncover non-substance addiction triggers inside and outside of your home.**
Not all addictions are tied to alcohol and drugs. Take time to track non-substance addictions tied to your environment. Does having a television in your bedroom make it easier to binge-watch Netflix until 3:00 a.m.? Does allowing social media alerts on your smartphone result in more online shopping? Look around your home and your neighborhood to identify addictive behaviors you want to change.

》 **Journal about your environmental triggers.**
Use your Substance Use Journal to identify ways in which your location triggers your substance use. Perhaps you find that you only drink alcohol in bars with your colleagues or usually smoke weed at a friend's house but never your own. Use that information to try to modify your usage pattern.

》 **Become environmentally aware outside of your own home.**
Have a conversation with someone else about how their environment has impacted their health. Ask them for three things that they feel support their health (like nearby parks) and three things that are detrimental (like nearby high-traffic roads). See if those influences apply to you and decide together how to lean into the good ones and overcome the potentially detrimental ones.

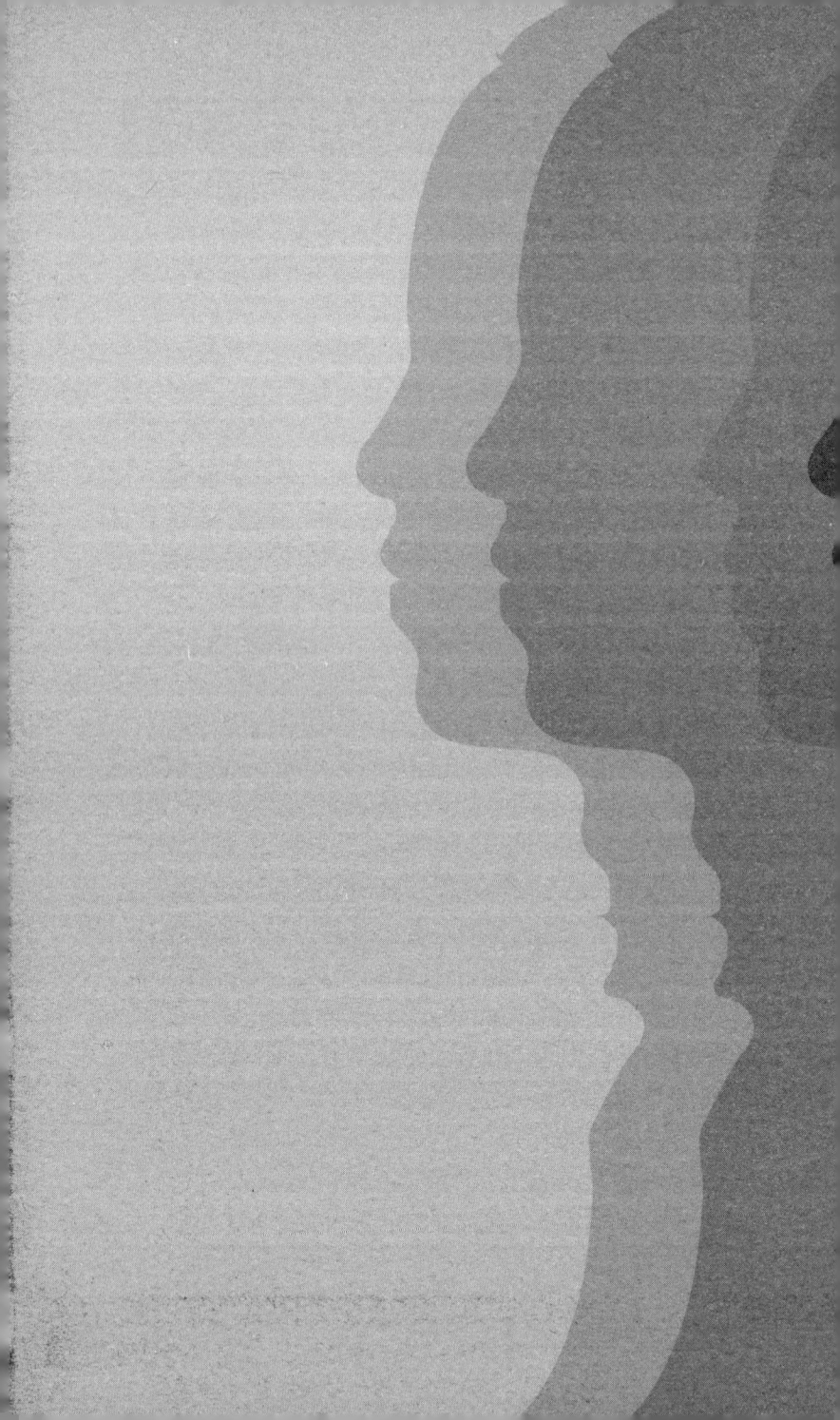

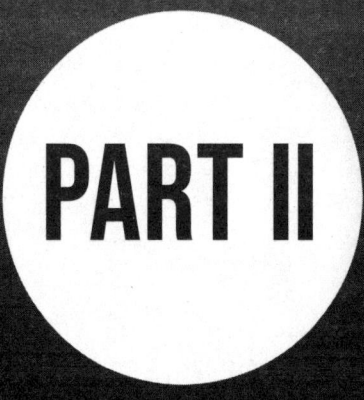

PART II

The Addiction Risks We Acquire

CHAPTER FOUR
Is Finding a Man the Solution for Jan?

Three prescription pills and one big problem

In 1970, if you were a doctor opening up the April issue of the *Archives of General Psychiatry*, immediately following the table of contents and long before you got to the article titled "Relationship Between Aggression and Depression," you'd come across an advertisement that looked like a retro Instagram grid to modern-day readers. Think of it as a #ThrowbackThursday. A way, way back Thursday. The old-fashioned-looking feed is a 3×3 grouping of images with muted color and black-and-white photos starting in 1955 and spanning fifteen years in the life of a woman named Jan. She's a slender blonde with a secret problem that only becomes apparent by the ninth and final picture, dated 1970.

In one photo marked 1959, there's a sporty shot of Joey with his left hand in his jeans pocket and his right hand on the hood of what looks like an old-school Chevy. He looks like he's been waxing that car to a shine all day so he can take Jan to the drive-in later. But maybe he got a little too frisky for her because we don't see him again. In 1961, at twenty-six years old, Jan has moved on and has one arm wrapped around Ted and the other around an oversized stuffed animal that Ted won for her in a carnival game. Behind them are endless rows of balloons, a few of which Ted, a bit of a Poindexter, may have popped to win her the prize. But it looks like Ted wasn't much of a prize because by the next photo, Jan has moved on again.

At twenty-nine, Jan and Charlie are taking in the sun and sand at the beach. Charlie seems a little wacky, with his zebra-print jacket. He stands proudly with a white dab of sunscreen on his nose (remember those days?) and a multicolored beach ball in the crook of his left arm. Jan sits with her legs to the side, modestly showing off her figure but not touching Charlie at all. Finally, it looks like New Year's has arrived and Jan has less than zero interest in a kiss at midnight. Her stocky date, Bunny, is sporting a suit, tie, and the perfunctory New Year's Eve cone hat. He looks plenty happy with a cocktail in his hand. But Jan looks like she'd like to be taken home. Immediately.

In between the boyfriend shots are photos of Jan with her father. In the story on the right page of the spread, we learn that Jan couldn't find a man because none of the guys she met over the years ever measured up to her tennis-playing, Scrabble-loving dad. The ninth and final picture I mentioned earlier shows Jan posing, alone, on a cruise ship. Her hair's a little messy, her tan coat doesn't betray a single curve, and her expression makes it seem like she wanted the photographer (perhaps the purser or concierge of the cruise ship) to take the damned photo already. Jan's pictures are next to a headline that reads: "35 and Single." The caption on the following page describes Jan as one of "the unmarrieds with low self-esteem." "Now she realizes she's in a losing

IS FINDING A MAN THE SOLUTION FOR JAN?

pattern—and that she may *never* marry." But there's one thing that could save Jan, the story hints. And that one thing is Valium (diazepam).

Jan was just looking for a man. But advertisements in medical journals were telling doctors to drug her up so what was casually called spinsterhood didn't depress her so much. Or so the pressures of motherhood or the frustrations of being a woman in the 1960s and '70s didn't upset her. At the time this classic advertisement debuted, Valium was part of a new class of drugs, benzodiazepines, that were gaining appeal and taking the market by storm. Other ads featured overworked and unpaid stay-at-home moms who were exhausted and unhappy running after their little ones. Or the shattered image of an anxious man with a red film over the picture. "Over the years, Valium has proven its value in the relief of psychoneurotic states—anxiety, apprehension, agitation, alone or with depressive symptoms," pharmaceutical company Roche boldly states in Jan's ad. "[It] can be a useful adjunct in the therapy of the tense, over anxious [*sic*] patient who has a neurotic sense of failure, guilt or loss."

But as Valium quickly became the top prescribed pill in America, concerns about the drug's safety began to rise. Overprescription was one concern. A 1979 *New York Times* article quoted a doctor testifying at a Senate hearing on the dangers of Valium: "Classically today, if a woman walks into her doctor's office and says, 'I'm nervous, my husband drinks too much,' the doctor will automatically give her a tranquilizer."

Within a decade of release, Valium became known as the "white-collar aspirin," "Mother's Little Helper," as the Rolling Stones called it in a song, and "Executive Excedrin." It wasn't just for the Jans of the world. In the 1970s, one survey found 15 percent of the population had taken

UN-ADDICTION

Valium or "one of its cousin drugs" in the past year. The other concern? Addiction. Valium is one of three highly addictive prescription drugs I'll tell you about in this chapter that you need to be wary of: benzodiazepines like Valium, opioids like Percocet (oxycodone containing acetaminophen), and stimulants like Ritalin (methylphenidate). (See summary on page 144.) Let's start with the first, Valium, that put the Jans of the world in an even more dangerous position than being single and childless.

Let's set aside, for a moment, the completely condescending, stereotypical take on Jan's life and the gross implication that a pill could get her the husband she needed to live a successful one. Even if, as a medical professional, you had the best of intentions to treat and manage anxiety that emerges in adulthood, if you did so with Valium, you might be loading one acquired biological risk (an addictive medicine) on top of another (anxiety). The story of Valium shows us how an acquired biological risk can come straight from your primary care physician.

When we talk about biological risk for addiction, we are not only referring to what is coded in our DNA (a factor we discussed in chapter one). Acquiring or developing a chronic illness may put a person on the path to addiction. You weren't born with insomnia but now you're awake staring at your clock until 3:00 a.m. every night. While there are less-addictive drugs currently used to treat insomnia, your doctor prescribes Valium, a drug sometimes still used to treat it. It may be decades since Jan was popping those pills—a quick fix for her spinsterhood anxiety—but the Valium prescribed today is the same old drug that it was back then, which means it carries the same addictive risks.

Taking a prescription pill can increase your chances of a substance use disorder. Though the medication is prescribed, it's in a class of medications, like benzodiazepines, stimulants, and opioids, that carry their own risk of addiction. While these two acquired biological risk factors often go hand in hand, they don't have to. The chronic illness can lead you to an addiction to a prescription drug or an addiction to a substance you're self-medicating with. At the same time, the prescription drug could be provided by a doctor, or it might come from a friend or through recreational use and leave you addicted. But that's not to say that Valium was an unnecessary or ineffective medication. In fact, it was extremely effective. Let me explain.

Benzos: False Hope of a Treatment for Anxiety Without Addiction

Benzodiazepines are used to treat anxiety and sleep disorders. Up to 40 percent of American adults report insomnia symptoms in a given year. On top of that, about one in three Americans (31.1 percent exactly) have or will experience an anxiety disorder at one point in their lives. We all know what it's like to stare at the ceiling until 5:00 a.m., but not everyone has experienced anxiety, so let's dive deeper. When we think about anxiety, we think about the ways it shows up in someone's life both physically and psychologically. Physically, it can elevate your heart rate, make your muscles tense, or cause your breathing to become shallow instead of slow and deep. That's your fight-or-flight response kicking in and preparing to get you out of danger. If you've got to run after that gazelle because you haven't eaten in weeks, you want your muscles ready to go. Psychologically, anxiety can make you feel irritable, tightly wound, or really nervous. Some people describe anxiety like having a round-the-clock soundtrack of that ominous music that plays right before something bad happens in a movie. The bad thing never happens but the music keeps playing and playing. Others think of it as the tiny first snowflake of thought that triggers an avalanche of worry over and over again. I tell my psychiatry students to imagine anxiety like a Ferrari going from zero to a hundred miles per hour down the autobahn of someone's emotional highway.

Benzodiazepines put the brakes on that Ferrari and slide it into park on the shoulder of the road. They do this by binding to the receptors in your brain that accept a chemical called GABA. Benzodiazepines have a very fast onset, some within a matter of minutes, so they're able to quickly create a sense of relaxation throughout your muscles and your mind. Back in the day they were sometimes referred to as "daytime tranquilizers." Some people describe Valium as simply helping them feel mellow or bringing them a much-needed calming wave. Others say it's euphoric, making them feel like they're a big marshmallow or as if they're lying on a cloud. It impacts the same part of your brain that alcohol does, so people often refer to it as a drink in a pill form. You don't have to suffer from anxiety to see some appeal there.

Other types of drugs with a slower onset (think extended releases) make it harder for your brain to connect taking the pill with finding relief. But benzodiazepines are quickly recognized and reinforced in your brain as something you need for an anxiety-free life. That leads to your prefrontal cortex to begin making a plan to ensure that you never go without that benzo, which brings us to our next problem: a benzodiazepine's offset. The drug can wear off so fast that it's like we're back in that Ferrari on the shoulder of the road, but we're going

IS FINDING A MAN THE SOLUTION FOR JAN?

from zero to a hundred again now that the anxiety is back. What people experience between doses is called rebound anxiety and is part of a withdrawal syndrome. That heart rate goes back up. That fear rises again. And the dopamine pathway says we need more benzodiazepine.

Another problem that pops up with benzodiazepines is growing tolerance to the drug. After months or years, one pill may not be enough for you and the dosage may need to increase to two. And, perhaps after that, three. This often happens with benzodiazepines, leading you to need more and more of the drug to get the same calming effect you did the first time. Put that on top of the rebound anxiety and you're having to use more of the drug to get the same effect and avoid withdrawal.

Ironically, benzodiazepines were heralded as the solution to relieving anxiety without addiction. The first benzodiazepine, Librium, was accidentally discovered in 1955 and marketed by 1960. It was quickly followed by Valium, which was released a year after a famous blond bombshell's death. In 1962, Marilyn Monroe was found facedown in bed, dead from an overdose. Among other medications on her bedside table was a newly filled prescription for Nembutal (a barbiturate) but the bottle was completely empty. Barbiturates, the class of drugs that preceded benzodiazepines, were known to lead to substance use disorders and even overdoses. But the pharmaceutical industry said that wouldn't be a problem with benzodiazepines. Plus, benzodiazepines were also an effective treatment for anxiety that hadn't responded to other medications in the past. Valium became the first $100 million brand the pharmaceutical industry had ever seen. So many millions of prescriptions were doled out that it was the best-selling medication in the United States between 1968 and 1982. Some experts think that the luster of Valium wore off when doctors started to see affluent White women falling victim to addiction. Others point to lawsuits and governmental regulations that made it harder to get the drug. But sixty years after its release, it seems as if everyone has forgotten the lessons in addiction that we learned about benzodiazepines. Because they're back—in fact, it's the second coming of the epidemic.

At this point, I should explain that Valium is the brand name of just one type of benzodiazepine. There are others that you may have also heard of including Ativan (lorazepam), Klonopin (clonazepam), Restoril (temazepam), and Xanax (alprazolam). And that last one I mentioned, Xanax, is the most dangerous benzodiazepine on the market. Here's why: Benzodiazepines are organized according to their half-life, which tells you how quickly they begin to wear off. Xanax leads the pack in terms of having the fastest onset and the fastest offset, making it the most worrisome. (You've just upgraded from that Ferrari to a Bugatti.) It drives addiction because it's so quickly absorbed into your system (think five minutes to relief) and then peaks at that half-life (around four hours) where you start to feel it wear off. You might not even be able to get through a night's sleep without waking up at 1:00 a.m. craving another pill. It's not hard at all to come by a prescription. Let me tell you about my patient Jack.

For Jack, his acquired biological risk skyrocketed on a trip to the ER. At twenty-one, Jack was preparing for midterm exams his junior year. He wasn't the first in his family to go to college, but he was planning to be the first to go to graduate school to become a lawyer. He'd

IS FINDING A MAN THE SOLUTION FOR JAN?

had weeks of late nights studying (and sometimes falling asleep) in the twenty-four-hour library on campus and meeting up with other students for study groups. He didn't give a second thought to the stress, even when he'd get sideways glances in the library from tapping his foot too loud or when he realized he'd spent more money on coffee than he had on food in the past month. "Hey, if this was easy, everyone would do it," he thought. But the night before his first final exam, he felt something he didn't expect. As he was studying questions from the previous year's exam, the words on the page started to come in and out of focus. It became harder and harder for him to breathe—almost like he had to force the air into his lungs—which was hard to do because there was also a terrifying pain in his chest. And he was shaking. All over. His uncle had had a heart attack a few years earlier, so he thought he knew the signs. Although he was dizzy, he made it to his roommate's door and asked him to help him get to the emergency room.

At the ER, Jack wasn't diagnosed with a heart attack. Instead, they informed him that he had a panic attack. (Here's your first biologically acquired risk factor: illness. An anxiety disorder.) They sent him home with a prescription for 1mg tablets of Xanax. (Here's your second acquired biological risk factor: a prescription medication that changes your biology.) Jack was supposed to take the Xanax, as needed, and was given instructions to follow up with his primary care physician. But he didn't have a PCP. What he did have were final exams to get through. And then a prestigious internship over the winter break. So, he took the Xanax to help with his stress going into an exam or cramming to write a paper, but the panic attacks kept happening. And he kept taking more and more pills—until he ran out after a month.

UN-ADDICTION

This is the part of the story where we hope that Jack would've gone to a doctor's office, but instead he ended up on Snapchat ordering some Zanzibars, a street name for Xanax which, shockingly, costs only a few bucks per "bar." A sophomore he'd seen before in one of his ethics classes would drop the package off at his dorm room. Weeks later, he was taking up to 8mg a day. That's eight times the amount that any doctor would prescribe. If he wasn't passed out from taking so much, he'd wake up in withdrawal and reach for a pill. Jack showed up at my office when his grades started slipping and friends started distancing themselves from him. "Xanax is the only thing that helps me with anxiety," he told me. We challenged that statement all the way to recovery. After sending Jack to an inpatient detox from the Xanax (yes, it's just that dangerous), I showed him how therapy, stress reduction, and a safe, nonaddictive medication like Zoloft could take its place.

Jack's story has been a common scenario over the past few decades By 2013, prescriptions for benzodiazepines were being handed out at the rate of 135 million per year. Over a seventeen-year period, the number of prescriptions had increased by 67 percent and the amount of those prescriptions was up by 300 percent. Unfortunately, the number of overdose deaths from the drug spiked as well, by a stunning 400+ percent. In 2007, you had Lil Wayne singing about mingling with the stars, throwing a party on Mars, and being a prisoner locked up behind Xanax bars. In 2012, our Brown bombshell, Whitney Houston, accidentally drowned in a bathtub with a mix of drugs, including Xanax, in her system.

The increase in benzodiazepine prescriptions in the 2000s may have led to an excess availability for another demographic of users beyond

IS FINDING A MAN THE SOLUTION FOR JAN?

those stressed-out older women targeted in the 1970s. Now teens were getting their hands on the drug. Despite the fact that, in 2016, the number of prescriptions was declining, the number of teenagers with substance use disorders related to benzodiazepines was on the rise. Whether they were sneaking them from medicine cabinets or buying them off social media, the perception may have been that taking a prescription drug was safer than an illicit one. That's not necessarily the case. And then came the pandemic. By March of 2020, anxiety and prescriptions for it were back on the rise and everyone from the FDA to scientists was sounding the alarm bell to try to avoid disaster.

Xanax marks the second coming of the benzodiazepine epidemic. But we can avoid it by asking our doctors those questions I'll outline at the end of this section. Because even though these drugs have a place in our collection of therapies to offer patients, they can also transform from being the solution to becoming the problem. That's exactly what happened with another drug class that has gotten a lot of press and also increases your risk of addiction: opioids.

Opioids: A Second False Hope of Pain Treatment Without Addiction

The story I shared about benzodiazepines probably sounded strangely familiar to the opioid crisis in America. Opioids were yet another prescription medication heralded by drug companies as not being addictive, but the reality was quite the opposite. Drug sales soared thanks to incentives being doled out to doctors to prescribe them. A new industry, the pain clinic, was born to keep a constant supply of the medication available. You weren't calling a drug dealer for opioids; you had a prescription. But it was still dangerous. And when prescriptions became too expensive or hard to come by, many people moved on to heroin. Roughly three out of four people who became addicted to illicit opioids (like heroin) started out taking prescription opioids. The problem wasn't just addiction; it was also overdosing. At the time of the writing of this book, ninety-one people die every day from an opioid overdose.

We often hear about opioids being prescribed for catastrophic accidents or end-stage illnesses like cancer. But you could end up with a bottle of opioids by just living your life. Delivered that baby by C-section? You might be sent home from the hospital with some Vicodin (hydrocodone containing acetaminophen). Or, maybe you recently retired and you're just trying to enjoy your golden years, but a little bit of pain is making it challenging to get around. For the elderly, dealing with the daily pain of arthritis could place a bottle of Percocet in the medicine cabinet.

I remember working as a consult liaison psychiatrist a few years ago in a hospital. I was sitting bedside with a young man whose sixty-eight-year-old father was exhibiting signs of delirium, not knowing what the date was, why he was in the hospital, or who his son was.

"Is your dad typically this confused?" I asked him.

"Only after he takes his medication," he responded.

We went down a list of all the prescriptions his father was on—five in total. On top of pills for high blood pressure, diabetes, and cholesterol, he was on Percocet (an opioid) for arthritis pain and Ativan (a benzodiazepine) for anxiety. Now this is one of the medication combinations I dread most. Both benzos and opioids suppress breathing, and taking the two together is a significant overdose risk—especially in

IS FINDING A MAN THE SOLUTION FOR JAN?

older adults. Increasing my concern even further, the son shared that although the benzo and opioid were only supposed to be taken as needed, his dad was taking them around the clock.

For all of you reading this who might be caring for aging parents, you'll see that it's not just important to make sure they're taking their medication as prescribed. You also need to know what medications they're on and what the risks of those medications might be. As we advance in age, our ability to tolerate drugs or strong medications of any kind declines. At the same time, the number of medications you're on also tends to increase.

This young man's dad may have been all right taking the two drugs separately on occasion, but when taken together, the drug-drug interaction (in addition to his age and lower tolerance) not only put him at serious risk for overdosing but was almost certainly the cause of his delirium. A younger person may have tolerated the drugs together and even increased their dosage. But an older person's brain has a harder time handling such potent medications. The result can be lightheadedness, confusion, or even becoming comatose. It took a week to taper the dad off Percocet and onto Tylenol safely because benzodiazepine withdrawal can be just as dangerous as usage. After a week, the delirium was gone.

One thing I need to drive home here is that it's not just the prescription that puts you at a higher risk for addiction. After all, we know that one in three American adults with arthritis filled an opioid prescription at a pharmacy in 2015. But less than 2 percent of Americans have a prescription opioid use disorder. It's the combination of biological, psychological, and environmental factors *plus* that prescription that pile up to push you over the edge to addiction. It could be an inherited risk that runs in your family. An ACE score of seven. A home address that puts a liquor store on every other block in your zip code. You and I could both get that prescription for an opioid after a surgery, but that doesn't mean we'll both end up buying heroin on the street when our prescription runs out.

Stimulants: A Third Slippery Slope

Last, but certainly not least, the third medication I want to highlight for you is stimulants. Stimulants work by binding to receptors in your brain that release our natural adrenaline. That release of natural adrenaline decreases hyperactivity, increases focus, and keeps us alert. Parents of children with ADHD often worry that their child will become addicted to stimulant medications, like Adderall (amphetamine, dextroamphetamine) or Ritalin (methylphenidate), but being prescribed a stimulant can actually prevent a future substance use disorder. I'll say that again: ADHD meds when used as prescribed to treat ADHD don't increase your risk of substance use disorder. In fact, research has shown the exact opposite—that by treating ADHD you can prevent a future substance use disorder. In many cases, the risk of having untreated ADHD outweighs the addictive risk of taking a stimulant to treat it.

That said, I must consider all of the biological, psychological, and environmental factors that we've discussed when I'm deciding whether or not to recommend Adderall or Ritalin. If you have a personal or family history of addiction, I'll likely recommend an alternative, nonaddictive ADHD medication like Wellbutrin (bupropion hydrochloride) or Strattera (atomoxetine). But if we determine that the other medications are not effective, or otherwise not a good fit, the decision to use a stimulant is appropriate. In that case, I'm keeping an eye out for red flags that stimulant misuse or addiction may be developing (like running out of your pills early or requesting frequent dose increases).

I'm keeping an eye out for those red flags because even though the stimulant overuse epidemic is less recognized, it's still on the rise and the consequences can be devastating. Besides the prescription medications I listed above, cocaine is also a stimulant. And while less than 2 percent of the population has used cocaine in the past year, I can virtually guarantee that almost every single person reading these words right now has used a stimulant in the past twelve months because caffeine is also a stimulant. Espresso shots, coffee, tea, chocolate, they all perk you up. The only difference is the order of magnitude.

Don't Ditch All Your Prescriptions

If you're suddenly suspicious of everything in your medicine cabinet, don't be. I've seen that kind of fear or suspiciousness of medications cause patients to make decisions that are detrimental to their health. I once had a patient who was literally running herself into the ground. She'd been a long-distance runner since high school, but now she was in her early thirties and the pounding of the pavement had taken a toll. She kept getting painful hip fractures from her ten-plus-mile runs but didn't want to hang up her sneakers. "If I don't run ten miles a day, I can't handle everything that goes on in my head," she told me. But the pain was so intense, she worked her way up to two bottles of alcohol a day rather than use the pain medicine her primary care physician

Triple Trouble: Drugs That Should Be on Your Radar

I've given you the back stories on what I consider to be the three most dangerous prescription drugs on the market right now. Think of this list when you're about to get that prescription from your physician and ask a lot of questions.

- **Benzodiazepines.** These antianxiety meds also help with sleep. They induce calm by slowing down everything in your brain and nervous system. Many of these drugs have generic names ending in "pam" like Valium (diazepam), Serax (oxazepam), and Ativan (lorazepam). There's also Xanax (alprazolam) and Librium (chlordiazepoxide), the benzo that started it all.

- **Opioids.** Opioids are also called painkillers and narcotics. They block pain signals (physical and emotional) from your brain to your body but also give you a rush of pleasure-inducing dopamine. Most of these generic medications end in "one" or "ine" like Vicodin (hydrocodone containing acetaminophen), OxyContin (oxycodone hydrochloride controlled-release tablets), Percocet (oxycodone containing acetaminophen), Dilaudid (hydromorphone), MS Contin (morphine sulfate controlled-release tablets), and codeine. Fentora (fentanyl) also falls into this class.

- **Stimulants.** These medications increase the levels of brain chemicals that help you focus and stay energized. Look for a generic medication that ends in "mine" and "date" like amphetamines: Adderall (amphetamine, dextroamphetamine), Concerta (methylphenidate

IS FINDING A MAN THE SOLUTION FOR JAN?

extended-release tablets), Dexedrine (dextroamphetamine), Focalin (dexmethylphenidate), Metadate (methylphenidate hydrochloride extended release), Methylin (methylphenidate hydrochloride), Ritalin (methylphenidate), or Desoxyn (methamphetamine).

These prescription medications tap some of the same parts of your brain as alcohol and illicit drugs. The calming effect that people get after taking benzodiazepines is very similar to what happens after you have a few glasses of wine or a shot of whiskey. That's because benzodiazepines hit the same GABA receptor in your brain that alcohol does. Opioids work in the same part of the brain that heroin does, which is why many people find themselves chasing the euphoria of pain pills. Stimulants work in the same part of your brain that cocaine and methamphetamine do, giving a jolt of energy and focus by releasing natural adrenaline. Just like alcohol, cocaine, or heroin, once your dopamine pathway realizes how necessary these medications are to survival, it can tell your prefrontal cortex to make a plan to never go without it—and that's where problems can begin.

recommended. "I don't want to get hooked on opioids or pain pills," she said. She wasn't wrong to worry about developing an addiction to pain pills, but as she soon found out, not treating your pain also increases your risk for addiction. Alcohol felt more acceptable because she didn't need a prescription and she could get it in most grocery stores. And it worked—until she became so hungover that she couldn't get up in the morning to drive her son to school.

Through counseling and scratching beneath the surface of her alcohol use disorder, we discovered that her drinking was a combination of treating the pain and grieving something she knew she was losing: her ability to run. I've taken care of a lot of people who couldn't quit a sport despite the physical consequences it brought them. A runner's high releases feel-good chemicals, just like opioids work the endorphin receptors in your brain. We worked together to overcome her addiction to alcohol and to running. That meant naltrexone for her alcohol use disorder, psychotherapy to address her emotional pain, and switching from running to rowing to avoid the microtraumas to her hips and avoid her physical pain.

The goal isn't to entirely avoid being on medication. Sometimes we need to be on a prescribed drug. And while your body adjusts to all drugs, that doesn't mean that all drugs are addictive. We know that blood pressure rises as we age, so many elderly people need to be on blood pressure medications. Our bodies adjust to being on these medicines. If we stop taking them, our blood pressure will go back up. That's another way of saying that you're going through withdrawal from that medication the same way that people go through withdrawal from alcohol in the form of a hangover or withdrawal from cocaine in wanting another

IS FINDING A MAN THE SOLUTION FOR JAN?

line. Your body is physically dependent on that medication, but you are not addicted to it. You're not going to lie about your blood pressure meds or take so much that you lose your job or it makes you sick. That's the difference when we think about what can happen with medications and drugs—like opioids, benzodiazepines, and stimulants—that are addictive. People lose their livelihoods and their lives over these medications. We have to know the risks of taking them and the measures around reducing those risks before we swallow that first pill.

Even when I prescribe insulin, I run the risk of your blood sugar dropping too low. So, I tell my patients what the signs of low blood sugar are and what to do if they happen. (In case you're curious, it's to drink a glass of orange juice immediately.) When I'm prescribing an opioid, stimulant, or benzodiazepine, it's not low blood sugar I'm warning of. It's development of an addiction.

Drug Testing *Before* You Take the Drug

The three medications that we look at in this chapter all have therapeutic benefits. There will always be times when using one of these prescriptions is appropriate. There will also be times when we want to avoid using a prescription because we can see how dangerous it is looking at your personal risk. To understand that risk, there's one more tool I want you to have in the tool kit you share with your doctor. It's called the ORT (the Opioid Risk Tool, see pages 148–149).

Previously, we talked about CAGE questions, which are a perfect tool for determining whether you already have a substance use disorder with alcohol or any other drug. The ORT is a commonly used and validated tool for predicting whether you are at increased risk for developing a substance use disorder if prescribed opioids, benzodiazepines, or stimulants, in particular. One reveals a substance use disorder, the other can prevent it. And, yes, even though it says "opioid," it actually works for all three classes of drugs.

Another key difference between CAGE and the ORT is that the latter takes two additional risk factors into account: your age (which we've talked about in this section) and any psychological conditions that might put you at risk (which we've also discussed in this section).

Unless you've seen a pain medicine specialist before, most of you will be reading and taking this test for the first time. Even if you've taken it before, go over it again. You may have been newly diagnosed with a mental health concern or learned more about your family history of substance use disorders after filling out your family tree. In the research study that validated this screener, 90 percent of people who scored eight or higher developed symptoms of opioid use disorder within one year of starting on the prescribed pain medication. If you score eight or higher, you want to be sure to share that information with your healthcare provider—especially if they're about to put you on an opioid, benzodiazepine, or stimulant.

What a Computer Card Game Teaches Us About Recovery

Unlike the inherited biological risk that your family passes along to you, acquired biological risk factors can change over time. Research shows us how with a gambling game that happens to have a trick. Just

IS FINDING A MAN THE SOLUTION FOR JAN?

Opioid/Benzo/Stimulant Risk Tool

Use this tool before beginning therapy with any opioid, benzodiazepine, or stimulant. A score of three or lower indicates low risk for substance use disorder. A score of four to seven indicates moderate risk for substance use disorder. A score of eight or higher indicates high risk for substance use disorder.

MARK EACH BOX THAT APPLIES	FEMALE	MALE
AGE IS BETWEEN 16 AND 45 YEARS	1	1
FAMILY HISTORY OF SUBSTANCE USE DISORDER		
Alcohol	1	3
Illegal drugs	2	3
Prescription drugs	4	4
PERSONAL HISTORY OF SUBSTANCE USE DISORDER		
Alcohol	3	3
Illegal drugs	4	4
Prescription drugs	5	5
HISTORY OF PREADOLESCENT SEXUAL ABUSE	3	0
PSYCHOLOGICAL DISEASE		
ADD, OCD, bipolar, schizophrenia	2	2
Depression	1	1
SCORING TOTALS		

Source: National Institute on Drug Abuse. https://nida.nih.gov/sites/default/files/opioidrisktool.pdf

a block shy of a Central Park meadow where New Yorkers sunbathe, toss Frisbees, and lay out picnic blankets with friends sits the Icahn School of Medicine at Mount Sinai. Inside the hallowed halls of this multimillion-dollar training, research, and patient care facility, several

UN-ADDICTION

researchers were in search of answers to a pressing question about cocaine use. If drug use damages the brain, could abstinence repair it and improve function in any way?

For six months, they followed over a dozen men and women with cocaine use disorder. After getting baseline data on the structures of their brains using MRI, they had the participants play a few games of skill. One that ended up being very telling: the Iowa Gambling Task.

When the computer screen comes to life, it looks like you've been transported back to the days of one-button joysticks and television screens with dials attached. Despite the throwback, the game is still enticing, and the rules are very simple. You start with a purse of $2,000 and the goal of winning as much money as possible by selecting cards from one of four piles. (Insert your own slot machine sound and flashing Vegas lights effects here.) Each time you use the computer's mouse to pick a card, you'll either win money, lose money, or break even.

At the start, it seems like a game of chance. But after a few rounds, participants may notice there's a pattern. Two of the decks always pay out a small amount ("You won $50!") or force you to break even ("You won $50! Fee of $50 applies."). The other two decks offer a big reward ("You won $100!") or a big loss ("You won $100! Fee of $250 applies.").

It's not hard to see which pile you should opt for. Slow and steady wins the race with the small payouts and small, occasional fees. But just because that's the logical choice doesn't mean that the thrill of a $100 payout is resistible. Indeed, many of the subjects opted to risk a whopping $250 fee for the possibility of $100. But that was when they were in a period of active drug use (though not under the influence at that moment in time). When the subjects, most of whom abstained

IS FINDING A MAN THE SOLUTION FOR JAN?

from drug use over the course of the six months, returned to retake the test, their scores soared higher. Less risky behavior. More cash in their computer game wallet. Why? They were able to make different, better decisions because their brains had changed.

Whether they completely abstained from drug use or significantly reduced usage, the volume of gray matter (cellular matter in your brain) increased in the long-term abstainers as did the structural integrity of their prefrontal cortex. That meant that their prefrontal cortex was better able to question the directives coming from the amygdala and motivation pathways. The players could take a moment and choose the slow and steady payout instead of the potential thrill of the $100 windfall.

Though the sample size was small, and the study was relatively short, the results were clear. Even though biology can put you at risk for addiction and drug use can impact your brain, it is possible for a person with addiction—and their brain—to recover.

So why aren't people getting the message? Because society's negative bias puts a tremendous amount of attention on relapse rates while more promising research and statistics get buried. Often, the focus is on the 25 percent of people with substance use disorders who do not recover. Which, of course, it needs to be, as that is too many of our loved ones lost to addiction. But what if I asked you to focus on the 75 percent of people with substance use disorders who recover? There are 20 million Americans in recovery. And part of that is thanks to the kind of biological changes that happen with abstinence.

Brain matter changes. Choices change. Futures change. It's incredibly hopeful news, rooted in the science of addiction. As amazing as that news is, I hope you're also thinking to yourself, "But what can be done to prevent getting to this point in the first place?" That all starts with the next sit-down I need you to schedule with your physician.

Mind-Changing Conversation #4: The Talk with Your Doctor

Protecting yourself from the acquired biological risk factors for substance use disorders means having more engaged conversations with the exact same professionals that you're already talking to about your acquired biological risk: your doctors. That's everyone from the primary care physician you have annual checkups with, to the dentist who is about to prescribe you oxycodone after your oral surgery, to the gynecologist treating you after a traumatic birth experience.

But before we jump into how to have those conversations, I have to let you in on two little secrets. First, most doctors don't get trained in substance use disorders. Unless you're speaking with an addiction medicine specialist or a pain management specialist, both of whom have had years of training in addiction, a conversation around decreasing your risk of a substance use disorder might be outside your usual MD's areas of expertise and experience. In that first conversation, your doctor might not have the ability to instantly give you the information, reassurance, and support you're looking for. Instead, I'm going to ask you to give your doctor something. Give them some grace and some space to get up to speed with you. One thing we are all taught in medical school is how to take a new set of information from a patient, jump into the medical literature, and come back to that patient with ideas

IS FINDING A MAN THE SOLUTION FOR JAN?

and guidance. So, expect, in all cases, that this won't just be a one-and-done conversation. It will be a continuing conversation with your medical professionals as you give them time to research and return to you with advice. And if you don't get a positive response or a return to the conversation, it's time to reconsider if this is the right doctor for you. It may seem extreme to switch doctors because of their views or lack of knowledge around addiction, but I'd say the same thing of any doctor for any other condition who wasn't able to provide the care you need.

You might've noticed that I said you need to continue the conversation with all your healthcare professionals, plural. That's because the second thing I want you to keep in mind is that you'll have to share this information with every professional who is part of your health journey. Due to federal laws currently in place, it is illegal for an addiction specialist, like me, to share your medical records with your primary care physicians, nurse practitioners, gynecologist, orthopedic surgeon, physical therapist, geriatrician, or any medical professional who could benefit from the information without specific, detailed consent forms allowing that communication. While these kinds of privacy protections definitely serve a purpose when you think about probation officers or law enforcement trying to gain access to medical records that could impact your life and livelihood, those same privacy protections can also become a frustrating hurdle to treatment or even dangerous to your health if we can't communicate with your other providers to coordinate care. For example, if I put a patient on propranolol (a nonaddictive medication known as a beta-blocker that helps with anxiety and also lowers blood pressure), I need to know if your primary care physician is managing your hypertension with another medication. That way we don't drive your pressure too low. If your physical therapist is helping you recover from knee replacement surgery, knowing that you have a history of substance use disorders and are taking opioids for pain could change their treatment plan. It might make them increase the frequency of your appointments so you get stronger faster and off the medication sooner.

You can do your part by being patient with your doctors and filling out all the forms, but also actively, verbally sharing information with all the healthcare professionals you meet with who need to be kept in the loop. Remember when we talked about being honest with your PCP? Even practicing what you'll say in the mirror? I know that having the same conversation repeatedly with all your doctors might feel annoying or even challenging right now. But imagine that repeating yourself is part of stigma reduction—because it is—and that change is starting with you. The more often you share this information with your doctors, the less awkward it will feel for you. Explaining how substance use disorder runs in your family or revealing that you have a substance use disorder will start to feel like telling your doctor that you have a history of diabetes or high cholesterol and are working to control it. But before I talk you through *what* to say, let's talk about *when* to say it.

Talk #1: "Can we talk about my risk of a substance use disorder?"

Before you send that email, sign on to that video call, or step into the office to talk to your doctor, you'll need to do some prep work. That starts with creating a comprehensive list of the different chronic illnesses that you have—diagnosed and undiagnosed. Write everything

IS FINDING A MAN THE SOLUTION FOR JAN?

down even if it doesn't seem like it could be a risk factor of substance use disorder. Because you never know. That chronic back pain that you're managing with Tylenol right now could progress to a point where you need something stronger to get out of bed in the morning. Or your hyperthyroidism might start to give you symptoms such as anxiety or mood swings that make you want to self-medicate with wine.

Once you have your list, start doing some research on whether these different ailments could be acquired biological risk factors for a substance use disorder. Hop on any search engine and ask, "Does chronic back pain cause addiction?" or "Can hyperthyroidism lead to substance use disorder?" Just make sure that you click on reputable sites like ones ending in .gov, .org, or .edu. (See pages 236–237 for suggestions on where to start your research.) And, in case you're curious, the answers to both of those hypothetical web searches above is yes.

One study of thousands of U.S. adults found that people with chronic lower back pain are more likely to have used meth and heroin in the past thirty days compared to adults without chronic lower back pain. Similar stats came up for increased usage of other drugs as well.

Another study looked at more than a thousand veterans to determine that patients diagnosed with hyperthyroidism had increased incidence of cocaine use disorder.

The next list you'll create is one of the prescription medications you're currently taking. Your job there is to see if there's a risk of addiction associated with that drug. You can look at the patient information pamphlet that comes with each refill or search for the information online. Remember, all drugs carry with them some negative side effects.

So don't panic if your search turns up a long list of side effects that concern you. I mean, we've all seen those television commercials for medications that race through a list of side effects while the actors happily kayak down a river. Just plan to talk to your doctor about it so the two of you can work together to consider the risk of your untreated illness versus the risk of the medication.

Finally, you're going to make a list of any risk factors that you've noticed after taking the Opioid Risk Tool for prescription drugs and the CAGE questionnaire for other substances that you might be taking. If you've been struggling with depression or gotten angry because someone approached you about cutting back on your alcohol use, there's no better time to start (or continue) that conversation with your doctor.

Once you get to the appointment, I want you to avoid using the following three words at all costs: "Google told me." If there's one thing that is super frustrating for doctors, it's when you reference your internet search as gospel. Remember, your healthcare relationship is a partnership between you and your doctor, which can be enriched by medical information for reliable sources on the web, as opposed to a relationship between you and Google, where you're just looping your physician in to follow Google's orders. When you approach your doctor, share with them what you've learned through your research, reveal what you need to tell them that you haven't talked about before, and request to discuss more in this visit or the next to reduce your risk. That might sound something like:

> Hi, Dr. Harrison! I read on a National Institutes of Health
> site that my fibromyalgia might be increasing my risk for a

IS FINDING A MAN THE SOLUTION FOR JAN?

substance use disorder. I took an Opioid Risk Tool assessment that I found online and had a low score. I also have a low ACE score. But I'm still concerned. I haven't told you this before, but my mother had an alcohol use disorder. In fact, in college, I stopped drinking because I worried I was getting drunk too often. I really want to make sure we're thinking about my risk in a way that's protective to me. On my next visit, can we talk about three or four specific steps I can take? And in the meantime, are there any resources you can point me to?

The beauty of this approach is that you're sharing information, building a partnership with your doctor, and giving them time to devise a smart strategy—if there's no sense of urgency. But what if there is a sense of urgency? Perhaps it's revealed that you're very worried about a drug you're currently on or you're already not taking that medication according to instructions. That might create an opportunity for another type of critical conversation.

Talk #2: "I'm worried about the drug or prescription medication I'm currently on."

Remember, this is a conversation where you share what you've learned through research, reveal what you need to tell them that you haven't mentioned before (including red flags), and let them know the support you need. For a prescription drug, that might sound like:

Hi, Dr. Harrison. I saw a study online about [insert drug here] that really worried me and I'd like to talk more about it with you. I haven't mentioned this before, but I've been taking more of the [insert drug here] than you prescribed. I even started borrowing pills from another friend who isn't using them. I thought about going to see another doctor to get an additional prescription last month—and I know that's a red flag. I'd really like to get off this medication before it becomes a problem. What can we start doing today to keep me safe?

You should know that hearing words like this is the best part of a doctor's day. In case you haven't heard, I'll let you in on another little secret: doctors feel pressure to prescribe medications. You might not be someone who does this, but there are countless Americans who come into their doctor's office looking for a pill to solve their problems—it's part of our culture! Fewer come in wanting to get off or reduce a medication. Asking us to help wean you off a medication that has a risk of addiction or reduce your exposure to it makes many of us absolutely thrilled.

Because of the urgency around a request like this, we have several strategies we can use to reduce your risk. For prescription drugs, that can include switching you to another medication that doesn't carry the same addictive risk (usually our first course of action), keeping you on the medication for the shortest time possible, or lowering the dose of the medication that you're currently on.

The entire risk mitigation plan shouldn't be biological, meaning it should address more than just what pill you're taking and when you're taking it. I also hope that your doctor considers leaning on psychological and social resources as well. Perhaps if they're worried about you taking

IS FINDING A MAN THE SOLUTION FOR JAN?

too much, you get a two-week supply instead of a thirty-day supply. Perhaps someone else in your home holds on to your medication for you or you keep it in a lockbox. Maybe you even request drug testing at appointments as a strategy for maintaining open, honest communication.

If the conversation you're having with your doctor is about nonprescription drug or alcohol use, that might sound like:

> Hi, Dr. Harrison! I saw some research online about how chronic lower back pain can increase my risk of addiction and I'm worried that's exactly what's happening with me. I started drinking more to deal with the pain but need to stay focused for my family and my job—and to be honest, my husband noticed and complained to me about it. I've thought about buying drugs off the street for the pain—but I don't want to do that. How can we get rid of this pain and this possible addiction?

I want to acknowledge that it's natural not to want to mention your drug use at all. In this book, I'm asking you to stretch beyond what feels natural and live in what is necessary for your health. Even if you can't stretch yourself all the way to the full story, stretch your way to start sharing the truth. Maybe, in the example above, you didn't just think about buying drugs off the street—you actually did. Getting halfway to the full story is better than not sharing the story at all. This might be the hardest, most vulnerable, and most important conversation you've ever had in your life. My hope is that you get the type of response that I offer to my patients. I tell them that I'm glad they trusted me with this information. I then guide them through an evaluation to determine how much of an impact the medication is having on their life. Finally, we talk about next steps based on what I find out. If you go to a doctor for diabetes concerns, they would check your vitals, test your blood sugar, and then talk about diet and exercise changes. If you're going to a doctor for addiction concerns, the visit will be similar. They'll likely check your vitals by looking for elevated blood pressure, and draw your blood to check for anemia, low Vitamin B, and liver or kidney damage. These are the types of changes that happen in your body as a result of harmful substance use. They'll give you some suggestions such as support groups, therapy, and medication recommendations.

Talk #3: "Before I fill this prescription, can we talk about this drug?"

It is so much easier for me to prevent you from getting on a dangerous medication in the first place than for me to help you get off of it once you've become addicted. I want you asking this question right after your doctor says, "I'm going to give you X medication." By the way, this is an excellent conversation to have for yourself or for a loved one or friend you're taking to the doctor. It might sound like:

> Hi, Dr. Harrison! I'm really glad my sister won't have to worry about being in really bad pain after her knee replacement surgery. I did want to ask a few questions about the medications you're putting her on before we fill the prescriptions. I feel like I've read something about the dangers of one of these drugs online and I should tell you, if she hasn't, that our brother has a substance use disorder. My questions are:

IS FINDING A MAN THE SOLUTION FOR JAN?

» **"What category does this drug fall into? Is it an opioid? A benzodiazepine? A stimulant?"** Use this information to start a conversation around what you've just learned about these drugs.

» **"Does this medication have any risk of addiction?"** If your doctor says yes, they might evaluate your risk using the Opioid Risk Tool or a lengthier assessment test. From there, you can talk about safety plans and alternative medications.

» **"Can we talk about the dose?"** It's worth asking if there are other things you can do that might reduce the dose of the medication you need or how long you need to be on it. Are there any life changes you can make that would decrease the dose you need? For example, if you did five minutes of deep breathing each morning, could that decrease the amount of Ativan you're taking?

» **"How long do I need to be on this drug?"** If you're concerned about the amount of time that your doctor anticipates, express your concern and ask if there are steps you can take to shorten the length of time you'll need to take the drug. Do the same if you start taking the drug and your doctor wants to increase your dose or doesn't take you off of it when your prescription is up. Revisit the conversation if you start taking the drug, get to the amount of time your doctor predicted, and your prescription is refilled at a higher dosage.

Un-Addicted: Your Acquired Biological Risk

Even if you've steered clear of street drugs your entire life and never taken more than two Tylenol for pain, this chapter has shown you ways you could still be at biological risk for addiction. You've just learned that certain prescription drugs are exponentially more powerful than willpower will ever be, that emotional and physical pain are potent forces, and that so many situations that put us at risk are beyond our control. Here are the points I want you to focus on.

Key Takeaways

» **Your risk of addiction is tied to biological changes that happen after birth.**
It's not just about your DNA. From diseases to injuries to prescription medications, your physiology can change over time and increase your susceptibility to addiction.

» **Three classes of Rx drugs are the most addictive.**
Review the summary on page 144 and commit to memory that benzodiazepines, stimulants, and opioids are the ones to watch out for. Knowing that is half the battle.

» **Anyone can be made vulnerable to addiction at any time.**
It doesn't matter if you're seventy-five with arthritis or twenty-five and have just gotten opioids for a broken collarbone. Addiction doesn't care about your age, race, gender, sexual orientation, or geography.

Your Homework

» **Start the conversation.**
Talk to your doctor about the potential addictive risk of any medications you already take or new medications they might prescribe. Be sure the two of you are on the same page about reducing your risk. And be sure to revisit the conversation if you start to notice you might be having early warning signs of addiction.

» **Advocate for someone else.**
If your parent, best friend, or neighbor has a health condition that might require one of the three drugs we talked about in this chapter—and you feel comfortable talking to them about it—let them know what you've learned and offer to go to an appointment with them to advocate on their behalf.

» **Update your Substance Use Journal to include prescriptions.**
Even if you're only taking them for a short period of time, include your prescriptions in your journal and watch for red flags like taking more than prescribed or feeling your dosage needs to be increased.

CHAPTER FIVE

How Weathering Any Storm Can Wither Your Health

Adversity increases your chances of chronic illness

In the winter of 1990, assistant professor Arline T. Geronimus arrived at her University of Michigan classroom to be confronted by a small sea of disappointed faces. Before she could launch into the lecture for her "Women's Health and the Timing of Reproduction" class, she had to hear about the lectures a small group of students had gotten from their parents. Their parents had been reading newspaper headlines about Geronimus. They weren't happy, and they weren't about to pay another cent for their kids to learn from someone with what they considered outrageous views. The students were sorry, but they had to drop her class.

Geronimus had spoken about her recent research on teen moms at the American Association for the Advancement of Science's annual meeting. Unlike other conferences she'd spoken at, this one was attended by a lot of journalists. So Geronimus was totally taken aback by the media maelstrom that ensued once reporters started digging

HOW WEATHERING ANY STORM CAN WITHER YOUR HEALTH

into the research she presented. What her study had found was that in poor rural and urban communities, teenage mothers had lower infant mortality rates than mothers in the same community in their twenties. Geronimus's data bucked the public health message of the time that teen pregnancy was universally catastrophic and to be avoided at all costs—and the media had a field day.

In Kansas, the *Salina Journal* ran a headline that read: "Study Finds Poor Teens Better Off with Babies." The *Chicago Sun-Times* chimed in with "Teen Pregnancy OK for Poor, Says Study." The *Washington Post* took things all the way to the hilt with an editorial entitled "Buying Into White Supremacy" that mentioned Geronimus and stated, "Black women weren't put on this Earth just to have babies—especially when near-babies themselves. The slave owner may have thought so. It now seems he's not alone." But the most memorable headline Geronimus recalls was one that aimed a misdirected stab at her right in the headline, reading, "Research Queen Says Let Them Have Babies."

Planned Parenthood, the Children's Defense Fund, and others were also discrediting her in the media and protesting against her outside of the conference where she spoke. Her research was throwing chillingly cold water on all the data they had on the perils of teen pregnancy. This little professor at the University of Michigan that few had heard of before was rapidly on her way to being labeled the biggest threat to youth in the country. Letters were sent to the head of her university asking them to fire her. Geronimus received death-threat phone calls at home. "We know where you live," they told her when she picked up the phone while alone with her one-year-old. "We're very close. We have Uzis."

UN-ADDICTION

Clearly, enrollment was the least of her worries, but Geronimus convinced her students to stay for a few more lectures. She restructured her syllabus to devote the next few classes to explaining how the media got her message all wrong. The thing is, she wasn't telling anyone when to start a family with her research. She was trying to draw attention to the fact that while society thought the big problem for the women in her study was just their low income or disinvested communities, the reality was something much more insidious and pervasive that resulted in better birth outcomes for teens than women in their early twenties. She came up with a name for this theory of accelerated poor health and aging due to adversity. She called it weathering.

There are two meanings of the word "weathering," which is exactly why Geronimus says that she chose it. You might imagine a rock at the edge of a cliff being perpetually hit by waves. It doesn't go anywhere; it weathers the waves and the storms. That's evident in us as human beings. We find coping mechanisms to be able to weather the metaphorical storms in our lives as well. Some are healthy (like meditation and therapy). Others are less so (like overeating or using drugs and alcohol). Weathering is also a term we use to describe a change in appearance over time. The rock at the edge of that cliff might look more worn or aged over time. This type of weathering is also evident in us as human beings. We show the effects of stress in our skin, our weight, our posture, our mood. The "waves" that crash up against us are stressors and traumas that can be emotional, financial, physical, racial, and more. Geronimus believed that these traumas changed our health. She believed that because the teens had experienced less weathering, they had better birth outcomes. She had data that showed

HOW WEATHERING ANY STORM CAN WITHER YOUR HEALTH

weathering *was* happening. She just didn't have the science to show *how* it happened.

Geronimus's theory of weathering was in search of science that hadn't yet come to light. It wasn't until nearly two decades later that scientists made discoveries that supported her theory of weathering. First came allostatic load, a term coined by neuroscientist Bruce McEwen and psychologist Eliot Stellar in 1993. Allostatic load is a way of measuring the amount of wear and tear that stress has on the body by looking at cortisol (your stress hormone) and epinephrine levels (natural adrenaline), blood pressure, resting blood pressure, and more. In one study using allostatic loads, Geronimus found that both poor and nonpoor Black women had the two highest allostatic load scores compared to their male or White counterparts. Race, and the adversity that comes with it, was the common denominator.

Years later in 2009, molecular biologist Elizabeth Blackburn was awarded a Nobel Prize for her discoveries around how telomeres function. Telomeres are often described as the protective caps on the end of DNA strands in your body. The shorter they are, the more you've aged. Telomere research had shown that White mothers of special needs children had shorter telomeres than those with children who did not have special needs.

Geronimus used this new science to show the impact of all types of adversity (poverty, race, lack of support systems) on different groups. With new metrics, Geronimus had a new path to persuasion. Her theory of weathering could become what is now accepted as fact by mainstream medicine. It's also what I turn to in order to explain what I'm teaching you about in this chapter: acquired psychological risk.

UN-ADDICTION

Let's take a moment to consider what happens when your body is under chronic stress. Geronimus looked at many different types of chronic stress, but let's focus on racism. We now know that racism isn't just a psychological trauma; it's also a physiological stressor. We can draw a straight line from racism to health disparities due to systemic failures, low socioeconomic status, lack of access, and more. One study of more than 330 Black teens in the rural South, for example, found that those who had experienced frequent racial discrimination without emotional support from parents (there's the power of PCEs again) had higher blood pressure levels and body mass index by age twenty. In just a matter of a few years, the trauma of having racial slurs hurled at them or being physically threatened had taken a toll.

When you experience racism, your body can have a physical reaction. Your mouth might get dry, your muscles can tense up, or you may start to cry. Your stomach could start churning. Your body could be propelling you into fight-or-flight mode. Is this going to escalate? How are you going to protect yourself? Do you need to get out of here? *Can* you get out of here? Maybe "here" is your job and you need the money. Maybe "here" is the home where your stepparent, who doesn't accept you, lives. What you're experiencing is a trauma response that can be triggered by everyday racism. When these things happen, they are threats not just to your self-worth but also to your ability to thrive or even stay alive. They trigger that dopamine pathway in your brain that says your survival is under attack. That level of discrimination is a trauma that you're enduring—and its impact can be brutal. Those tense muscles? That can lead to back pain and heart attacks. Those cortisol rushes for fight-or-flight? That can lead to spikes in blood sugar, increased cholesterol, and heart disease. All of these things prematurely age you, which is exactly what Geronimus found. And all of them can increase your risk of a substance use disorder.

When Trauma Looks Like Breaking Through a Concrete Roof

We've all heard of the proverbial glass ceiling in the workplace. That barrier for women in corporate America that allows us to see the success happening in the upper rungs of the corporate ladder, but prevents us from obtaining those titles, salaries, and leadership roles without some Herculean force to shatter the glass and get to the other side. Now imagine for a moment that, as a Black person, trans person, immigrant, or member of another marginalized community, instead of chipping away at that proverbial glass ceiling in the workplace, it felt more like you were trying to punch your way through a concrete roof. Every effort of applying for those promotions is physically and emotionally exhausting. Never being sure if you could actually make it to the other side but throwing those punches anyway. Not being at the dinner parties, in the meetings, or on the golf course to get a look at the other side of that concrete roof to help you decide if it was what you even wanted.

Or worse, imagine that instead of a glass ceiling or concrete roof, it's what some experts call a "glass cliff" that you're being led over and off. That you are ushered forward on a path you deserve but aren't given the support you need. Or you're given a promotion simply for the sake of company optics—a promotion that sets you up to fail. In any of these situations, once you've "broken through," you're still dealing with the constant pressures of being "The One" or "The Only." Absorbing all the pressures of existing in a space not as a person, which of course we all are, but as *the* Black person on staff or *the* trans person at the company. On top of all the pressure of your new position comes the pressure of representing all the women, all the Black people, or all the trans people. It's an impossible job, an unfair job to be given, but you have to do it under a spotlight and surrounded by people who don't necessarily understand who you are, where you're coming from, the monumental task you've been given, or the steep implications of not succeeding. And eventually, it may turn out that the glass ceiling is not the only thing that has been broken, as you start to buckle under the pressure.

When human beings need a quick fix in our lives, we often turn to substances. This is one of those situations. Substances to help us cope with the occasional bad day at work, difficult conversation with a boss, or tough break on a promotion. In fact, at least in the U.S., this is a very prominent part of culture. It's five o'clock somewhere, right?! But what if those things happened not just occasionally or once a day? What if they happened multiple times per day? When you think about that concrete ceiling or that glass cliff, you can imagine an urge to turn to those coping mechanisms much more frequently than any of us might want. After months of stress brought on by subtle, indirect, and even unintentional racism (also known as microaggressions), that's exactly what happened to a Black colleague of mine who was The Only Black Person in a senior management position at her company a few years ago.

When she reached out to tell me how much she was struggling, her experiences sounded all too familiar. She'd be in meetings where her

HOW WEATHERING ANY STORM CAN WITHER YOUR HEALTH

colleagues loudly complained that they couldn't find any minority candidates for senior positions—but would easily find them for lower-paying support positions. The only people she saw who looked like her worked in reception or janitorial positions. Her capabilities were constantly questioned, whether it was about her being the lead presenter for a pitch to a new client or offering an innovative approach to solve a problem. ("No thanks, that's not how we do things around here" was usually the reply.) And then there was the time when she proudly told a colleague that her son was accepted at an HBCU (Historically Black College or University). "Why would anyone choose an HBCU over Harvard?" the woman asked.

What she absolutely couldn't stand at all were the everyday passive-aggressive questions about Black culture and current events that could just as easily have been answered by doing a Google search, listening to a *Red Table Talk*, or reading a think piece in *The Atlantic*. She needed to find a way to take the edge off. Not that it was hard doing her job, but it was hard doing her job plus being the Michelle Obama of her office—never getting angry, always being pleasant, always with a smile despite the micro- and macroaggressions. I saw an amazing video as part of our cultural sensitivity training at Eleanor Health and have been using it to describe these aggressions to other folks ever since. The video said to think of these micro-insults as mosquito bites. It's annoying but tolerable when you just get one. But imagine if you got one, two, or three every day at work. By the end of the week, those mosquito bites would be overwhelming. By the end of the month, you'd be looking for another job—if only it were that easy—because the job you have is infested with mosquitos and you're being sucked dry.

UN-ADDICTION

For many different reasons, my colleague couldn't leave her job. She had worked extraordinarily hard to climb the corporate ladder so high and positions like hers were not easy to come by. She also hated the idea of being chased out of her ideal job. Why should she spend her free time sending out résumés and making up excuses to go on interviews when she actually loved the work she was doing? Her coping mechanisms started with an occasional drink at the end of her day to shake off the frustrations of her job and enjoy time with her family at night. An occasional drink at the end of the day turned into an occasional drink at lunch so that a tough morning at work wouldn't lead to her "popping off" at her coworkers later that afternoon. It was a few ounces of prevention against the catastrophic consequences such a pop-off could cause her professionally. But it wasn't working. Instead of lashing back at her coworkers, she started having panic attacks in her office before meetings or after she was done holding it together at a work event.

By the time she reached out to me, her job wasn't in jeopardy but her mental health and her personal life most certainly were. Her husband and kids only got to spend time with the intoxicated version of her and she felt like she was constantly in fight-or-flight mode, unable to find a state of calm. I could draw a straight line from the trauma of the discrimination and racism she was experiencing at work—these acquired psychological risk factors—to her substance use. "I have to drink to tolerate these people at work," she told me.

She truly felt like her only options were to drink or to quit her job. Luckily, we found her a better solution. We talked about the first step—recognizing we have a problem. In this case, the problem was the trauma of racism and discrimination, and its physical and emotional consequences. In her case, panic attacks and risky alcohol use. Once we identified the problem, we were able to think through possible solutions. I connected her with a Black woman therapist who was skilled in addressing the mental health impact of racism, so that she could share freely.

Having a culturally informed therapist who could understand her life experience meant that she had a safe space to step into during sessions where she wasn't under scrutiny and didn't have to worry about her experiences being questioned or invalidated. Just being able to talk about her experiences, uncensored, with a professional was a big relief. She also got tools for managing the experience she was having at work. She was diagnosed with anxiety and started on a medication that she could take instead of alcohol and eliminate those panic attacks. Her drinking came back down to unproblematic levels and she was able to show up more confidently in the workplace. It was the ideal resolution to the situation.

When Less Use Equals Higher Consequences

While research has found that racism can lead to increased substance use, I want to be clear that people of color don't have higher rates of substance use across the board compared to Whites. I'll say this again because it's a fact that is often misrepresented in medical literature, on television, in movies, and everywhere else you can think of. Contrary to popular belief, Black and Brown people aren't universally using substances with a greater frequency or experiencing substance use disorders in greater numbers than White populations. I've got the numbers for you to back that up, too. In the past year, 70.3 percent of Whites drank compared to 58.7 percent of Hispanics, 56.8 percent of Blacks, and 53.2 percent of American Indian or Alaska Natives. In the past year it was 0.7 percent of Whites who had used methamphetamine compared to 0.6 percent of Hispanics and 0.2 percent of Blacks. And when you look at overall rates of substance use disorders—including alcohol, prescription medications, and illicit drugs—7.8 percent of White people were dealing with these compared to 7.1 percent of Blacks, 7.1 percent of Hispanics, and 4.1 percent of Asians.

But here's the twist. While people of color don't have higher rates of substance use or substance use disorders across the board, they are more likely to experience the negative consequences of that use or disorder. If you're wondering how that can be, first know that it's not only the case for substance use disorders. For example, while Black women are 4 percent *less likely* to develop breast cancer, they have a 40 percent *higher* rate of death from the disease compared to White women. On that same note, while Blacks have a far lower incidence rate of skin cancer than Whites, we also have a much lower five-year survival rate. And like breast cancer and skin cancer, Black people have lower rates of substance use disorders overall, but once we have a substance use disorder, we're more likely to lose our job as a result of it or go to prison because of it, more likely to acquire another disease like cirrhosis of the liver, and even more likely to die from it.

This disparity in consequences with substance use disorder occurs for the same reason it does with other chronic illnesses. First, think about access to care. Marginalized communities are more likely to have trouble getting access to care or treatment for a substance use

HOW WEATHERING ANY STORM CAN WITHER YOUR HEALTH

disorder. On top of that, when you consider the most effective forms of treatment for substance use disorders, access is even more restricted. It's commonly acknowledged that the most effective treatment programs for substance use disorders are company-sponsored and exclusive to certain industries, like pilots, lawyers, nurses, and, yes, doctors. Physicians, for example, who go into profession-related recovery programs have a significantly lower risk of relapse with 71 percent being sober after five years compared to only 49 percent of the general population. But only 5.8 percent of doctors are Hispanic, and 5.7 percent of doctors are Black. Similarly, less than 7 percent of pilots identify as Hispanic or Latino, a little more than 4 percent are Asian, and less than 3 percent are Black. Like so many chronic illnesses in this country, your chance of managing or overcoming substance use disorder depends on your job and your access to care. Imagine wondering if a loved one you lost to a substance use disorder might still be alive if only they'd been a registered nurse instead of a nurse's aide or a pilot instead of a taxi driver.

Even once you do have access to care, you might be in a setting where you are repeatedly subjected to the mosquito-bite-like annoyance of microaggression or blatant racism. Both implicit biases (tied to our unintentional and unconscious judgments and stereotypical beliefs) and explicit biases (conscious and explicit displays of prejudice) show up in medical establishments. A 2005 study of hundreds of patients showed that even when Blacks had much higher pain scores, they were less likely than Whites to be given opioid painkillers. Another study similarly showed that physicians are twice as likely to underestimate the pain of Black patients compared to all other ethnicities combined. One possible reason, supported by existing studies, is that White medical professionals believe Black people experience less pain. Wondering why that would be the case? Starting back in the 1800s, physicians and scientists asserted that Black people were biologically closer to apes, while White people were more evolved. Along with this came a set of biological differences—one of which was pain tolerance. This belief has persisted. Highly educated professionals, like doctors, often think their educational level reduces implicit bias. That's not the case—and not recognizing this is dangerous. While we've seen decreases in explicit racism in medicine, we have not yet begun to see meaningful decreases in implicit bias—and this is why we continue to see these disparities.

These kinds of biases show up in addiction treatment programs across the country as well. Early in my career, I was a psychiatrist at an addiction treatment program where I saw this playing out firsthand. There was a clear difference in how the White staff described our White patients and patients of color during team meetings. Disproportionately, the White staff would call out Black men and women in the program as being "unmotivated," "noncompliant," and "resistant." They would excessively flag Black patients as being "not ready for recovery" and recommend them for discharge from the program. But White patients were called "depressed" and "anxious" and recommended for more intensive services.

I don't believe the White staff was racist. But they were very likely susceptible to the messages about Black people that can become programmed into all of us from television, movies, the news, and other media where Black people are portrayed as aggressive, angry, and uncooperative. I'm also sure that some of those Black patients didn't react well to having a White person in a position of power telling them "Take this pill or else" or "Show up for therapy or you'll get kicked out of here." I'm sure some Black patients did express anger in group therapy while processing their emotions, and I'm sure some White staff found it "threatening" and wondered if it was safe for those patients to be in the program. I wouldn't be surprised to hear that when White patients expressed the same level of anger, they were noted by White staff as having "decreased distress tolerance" and needing "coping skill development." That subtle racism had the power to rob patients of color of their right to effective substance use disorder treatment, so in my time at that clinic I worked hard to implement strategies to educate the staff and eliminate the disparity.

Complexities of Identities

I've been focused on highlighting the impact of racism, but weathering and the health impact of being discriminated against aren't only about race. The same parallels can be drawn whether we're discussing people experiencing discrimination due to their gender, sexuality, social status, or something else. The thread that moves through all the ways by which we identify people is that they are choiceless states. No one chooses to be Black, Hispanic, lesbian, or trans (or all of the above!). It's simply who we are. But these identities that define us to the core are often the reasons that so many people in America experience discrimination and adversity. When oppression, marginalization, and racism decrease, so do adverse effects like the risk of harmful substance use.

At the same time, beneficial effects, like positive identity and self-esteem, increase. Let's take a closer look at what's happening beneath the surface.

Listen to any expert talking about health disparities in America and they may eventually present the acronym REaLS to you. It stands for Race, Ethnicity, Language, and Sexuality. Within the healthcare industry, REaLS is a framework we use to evaluate different demographic groups so that we can watch for health disparities. Race refers to inherited physical characteristics used to describe people. You might call someone Black, Asian, or White because of how they appear. And you might also be dead wrong.

I'll never forget a telehealth session that I had with a patient during the pandemic. He was giving me a bit of a Willie Nelson vibe. He was in his sixties, looked White, and was a painter from the Midwest. We were meeting because of his marijuana and methamphetamine use disorder.

During our session, I started looking for adverse and positive childhood experiences by asking him to tell me about his earliest memories. It was a broad question that led to a bull's-eye moment. He told me that he grew up in a tiny, lily-white town in Iowa where all the kids called him a "porch monkey" because of his dark skin. I was absolutely stunned by the slur. As it turned out, he had a mixed background and wasn't blond-haired, blue-eyed, and pale-skinned like everyone else in town. He had a slight tan and darker features. He drew a direct line from those racial slurs and ostracism and started smoking cigarettes when he was just ten years old, began drinking alcohol before middle school, and first tried meth by the age of thirteen. It reminded me that you can truly never tell someone's experience (or race!) just by looking

HOW WEATHERING ANY STORM CAN WITHER YOUR HEALTH

at them. To my biased eyes, he appeared White, and I never would have thought being called porch monkey, a slur I thought was reserved for Black people, would ever be part of his ACEs. And yet, that experience carved a straight path to addiction for him.

Unlike Race, Ethnicity refers to acquired (not inherited) characteristics used to describe people, like a shared culture or language. Your race might be White (like the painter I just told you about) but your ethnicity could be Italian or Greek or Spanish. You might be Black, but your ethnicity is Jamaican or Cuban. Language is exactly that—the language(s) a person writes and speaks so that healthcare providers can make sure that they're able to communicate effectively. And Sexuality or sexual orientation refers to who you are romantically or physically attracted to. For example, are you asexual, gay, lesbian, bisexual, pansexual, heterosexual, or none of the above?

While REaLS is an important tool for noticing the most common ways in which we discriminate against and marginalize people in society, it's also an incomplete one. I know that it's impossible to capture all the infinite ways that people are discriminated against due to some aspect of their identity. I've even seen other experts transform REaLS to REALD to include people with disabilities. Others place an emphasis on Age as they analyze data. Ultimately, we could have an acronym with an alphabet soup full of letters to account for the myriad ways that sneaky little culprit of discrimination negatively impacts our health.

But I think one missing letter ("G" for "Gender Identity") is absolutely essential to looking at health disparities. So, at Eleanor Health and when I give presentations, I coined the phrase and talk about REGaLS (Race, Ethnicity, Gender Identity, Language, Sexuality).

Gender Identity is how you identify in terms of gender, whether that's male, female, neither, both, or somewhere in between. It isn't outwardly visible unless someone has updated their Zoom with their pronouns. When you look at the world through the lens of REGaLS, you can see people who may suffer endless microaggressions at their job because of their race, be harassed by their neighbors because of their sexuality, or be ridiculed by strangers because English is not their first language. All these experiences with racism and discrimination can result in a trauma reaction.

This is where the three Es of trauma-informed care come in: Event(s), Experience, and Effect. In my field, we use the three Es to help us identify and properly approach someone who has been through a trauma. First, we figure out the *Event* or series of events that were the source of the trauma. We recognize these as *Experiences* that lead to harmful psychological and physical impacts. Then we seek to uncover the *Effect* of those experiences on a person's physical or social well-being. Once you start practicing looking at the world through the lens of REGaLS, you'll begin to see the events, experiences, and effect of discrimination more often and more clearly. You'll recognize how an asexual person might have a different experience at the gynecologist's office than a heterosexual person. Or how a Black person might have a different experience at a cancer center than a White person. You'll begin to connect the dots to how those different experiences can lead to detrimental effects.

REGaLS and the three Es will also help you avoid invalidating an experience of discrimination that you or someone else has. When you or a loved one experiences a microaggression it's easy to think, "Did that just happen?" or "They probably didn't mean it." You can go through

HOW WEATHERING ANY STORM CAN WITHER YOUR HEALTH

a negative feedback loop invalidating your reaction to the experience you just had. Unfortunately, that's one of the biggest ways we worsen the impact of that trauma: by invalidating the experience entirely or denying that a trauma even happened. The three Es validate and bring attention to an event instead of bypassing it like so many of us do.

Years ago, my father was in the supermarket checkout line buying some groceries. He handed the cash over to the White clerk, who put his change on the conveyor belt. He was outraged by the slight. Why wouldn't the clerk put the money directly into his hand the way he had done for her? Was she determined to disrespect him? Did she not even want to risk touching him? Or was she moving so quickly toward bagging his groceries that she accidentally slighted him?

None of the answers to these questions matter, first of all, because we'll never really know; but second of all, because, to my dad, the clerk had clearly disrespected him because he was Black. Perception is reality here. What matters most in those moments is what you've perceived to happen and the impact it has on you. Whether the clerk meant to slight my dad or not, he felt slighted, and his fight-or-flight reaction was triggered. The damage was already done.

When you or someone else experiences a microaggression there can also be a tendency to overcompensate for the slight—something called John Henryism. As the folk songs and myths written about him go, John Henry was a Black steel driver who worked on building the Chesapeake and Ohio (C&O) Railway in the 1800s. He's mythologized as being the strongest man alive and the fastest with a sledgehammer—so strong and so fast that he takes on the challenge of competing with a steam drill (a new invention at the time) to see who could crush more rock.

Henry ends up winning the competition but dies from exhaustion at the end of it.

One of the morals of the story is around the tremendous effort Blacks frequently feel they must put in to be accepted in society—and how that effort can ultimately lead to us working ourselves to death. It's easy to think of reactions to microaggressions hundreds of years later in the same way. Perhaps the woman who is questioned about what's under her hijab becomes overly polite and explains everything she's wearing and how it's put on. Or the guy at the buffet signs up for an expensive gym membership after work and puts himself on a no-carb diet after being asked, "Are you sure you should be eating that?" Traumas can be insidious and have a long trail when it comes to the physical and emotional impact they can have on us. That makes identifying them even more important. Luckily, there is an easy way to do just that in less than five minutes.

What's Your Everyday Discrimination Score?

For decades, there has been a way to quantify how much discrimination you're experiencing so that you're aware and your doctor can factor it into your healthcare plan. It was developed in the nineties by David R. Williams, a graduate school professor of public health at Harvard University. But every time I show the Everyday Discrimination Scale (EDS) to other healthcare professionals, I'm met with shock. "Why have I never heard of this?" they ask me. "Why isn't this part of my education?" I'm sharing this with you in case that's the reaction that your doctor has when you show them your results. Don't be alarmed.

HOW WEATHERING ANY STORM CAN WITHER YOUR HEALTH

It doesn't mean your doctor doesn't care or that they're not a good physician—it just means this literally isn't part of our education (sadly!). Share with your doctor that you read about this scale in a book and that you'd like to talk about your results at your next appointment.

If your healthcare provider dismisses it or they aren't willing to discuss it, that's a sign you might need another provider. But chances are they'll approach you with curiosity and help you devise a more customized health plan. The beauty of the EDS is that it invites a conversation. I may find out that you've felt traumatized by a recent police shooting of an unarmed Black man on the news and that's resulted in you using substances more. That trauma and stress may be impacting your sleep, your immune system, and your support system. Maybe you're having more arguments with your partner and that's causing depression. Now I'm not just writing you a prescription for your annual mammogram or a Z-Pak to cure your cough and shortness of breath from the bronchitis you came in here with. I'm validating your experiences. I'm connecting you to a support system. I'm helping you recognize the connection between the discrimination you face and your substance use.

In general, the higher your score or frequency of occurrence, the higher your risk and the more it needs to be a part of your healthcare discussion.

Cultural Relevance as the Antidote to Inadequate Healthcare

With nearly everyone alive in the world today experiencing discrimination, the question isn't how to avoid it but how to fortify ourselves

The Everyday Discrimination Scale

For each of the following questions, answer:

Almost every day
At least once a week
A few times a month
A few times a year
Less than once a year
Never

Questions:
In your day-to-day life, how often do any of the following things happen to you?

1. You are treated with less courtesy than other people.
2. You are treated with less respect than other people.
3. You receive poorer service than other people at restaurants or stores.
4. People act as if they think you are not smart.
5. People act as if they are afraid of you.
6. People act as if they think you are dishonest.
7. People act as if they're better than you.
8. You are called names or insulted.
9. You are threatened or harassed.

HOW WEATHERING ANY STORM CAN WITHER YOUR HEALTH

If you answered "A few times a year" or more frequently to at least one question, also describe what you think is the main reason(s) for these experiences?

1. Your ancestry or national origins
2. Your gender
3. Your race
4. Your age
5. Your religion
6. Your height
7. Your weight
8. Some other aspect of your physical appearance
9. Your sexual orientation
10. Your education or income level

OTHER POSSIBLE CATEGORIES TO CONSIDER

1. A physical disability
2. Your shade of skin color
3. Your tribe

Other (SPECIFY) _____

Source: "Everyday Discrimination Scale." David R. Williams, graduate school professor of public health at Harvard University. https://scholar.harvard.edu/david rwilliams/node/32397

against those experiences and position ourselves to thrive nonetheless. In the same way that being silent about substance use disorders increases stigma around them, being silent about discrimination increases the power it has over those who are discriminated against. We must address discrimination if we want a better chance at health, happiness, and recovery. One of the ways in which we can do this for ourselves and others is by seeking out culturally relevant care. This might come from doctors, therapists, or healthcare providers that share an understanding of the REGaLS that you or your loved one identifies with. If you're a Black woman, you could seek out a Black primary care physician. If you have a trans male friend, you can research and try to find your friend a trans male therapist. With the rise of telehealth, the likelihood of getting at least online access to culturally relevant care has increased. You can also help your loved one come up with a list of questions they can ask the provider when they meet with them. For example, "Have you had cultural sensitivity training?" or "Is anyone on your staff bilingual?" or "How would you include aspects of my race, ethnicity, gender identity, sexual orientation, disability, age, or faith in my care?"

As much as we're trying to spend less time on our phones and tablets, mobile devices can provide culturally relevant care as well. Clinical psychologist Natalie N. Watson-Singleton developed a mindfulness app specifically for African Americans called Mindful You. Then she enrolled several dozen Blacks in a research study to use it. The for-us, by-us mobile health app contained distinctively African American design elements, including use of a logo echoing colors in African flags (red, green, yellow, and black); photos, illustrations, and animations exclusively of Blacks; and meditation practices that speak to the Black

HOW WEATHERING ANY STORM CAN WITHER YOUR HEALTH

experience, like "I Can Breathe" and "Cherishing Safety." Meditations were voiced by African American actors, rather than having, say, White actors telling Black listeners to know their worth or follow their lead. By the end of her small, two-week study, she found that stress levels had decreased for app users and the ability to emotionally regulate had increased. So did levels of self-efficacy around how to manage that ever-pervasive stress in the Black community.

I know we've been dealing with a lot of acronyms lately, but stick with me on this last one because it's going to pull everything we've been discussing together. In my field, we help people overcome substance use disorders with a trauma-informed approach that highlights the four Rs of trauma. You can use these four Rs in your own life to increase the compassion, understanding, and effectiveness of how you approach anyone who has gone through a trauma—whether it's a microaggression at work, an experience with intimate partner violence, a shouting match at a restaurant, or an uncomfortable moment at home. The four Rs are Realization, Recognition, Responding, and Resisting re-traumatization. So far, we've already tackled two of these Rs in the chapter. You now *Realize* the widespread impact that trauma can have on the people you interact with every day. You can use the lens of REGaLS to look at your partner, your child, your boss, your delivery guy, your bus driver, and anyone else in a new light. We've stopped asking "What's wrong with you?" and progressed to "What happened to you?" and even now: "Who hurt you?"

Recognition is about learning the signs and symptoms of what reacting to that trauma looks like. You've already learned that while it can frequently look like a substance use disorder, it also often looks like other health disparities we keep coming back to that are associated with hypertension, diabetes, or asthma. And guess what, it can also look like angry, aggressive, or uncooperative. *Responding* is one of those mind-changing conversations that you'll be able to have by the end of this chapter.

The last R is for *Resisting re-traumatization*, which we talk about above. None of us would actively seek to re-traumatize someone. It's often simply an accident. You let something slip like, "I can't stand it when women in domestic violence relationships don't leave. If that was me, I'd leave." That's re-traumatizing for anyone within earshot who has been in a domestic violence situation. Or if someone has a family member who dies of an opioid overdose and you accidentally say, "That would never happen in my family and if it did, I wouldn't tell anyone." Accidents happen. You can try to avoid them by recognizing, realizing, and responding; by choosing your words carefully; and by being aware of the blind spots we all may have. When we do re-traumatize someone, we can call ourselves out, receive it gracefully if someone else mentions it to us, validate them, take full responsibility for learning, and try not to repeat the same mistakes.

Now that you understand the complexities of identity, let's talk about the role you can play in supporting someone who may or may not identify the same way you do.

Mind-Changing Conversation #5: The Safe Space Talk

Discrimination is one of the chilling ways we kick people out of the pack. It denies you that dopamine trigger and survival signal in your brain that come from connection. But even in a world rife with discrimination, you can rightfully reclaim your pack status and the emotional boost it brings by intentionally pursuing a sense of belonging in your life.

One of the ways you can increase a sense of belonging is by locating and becoming a part of a safe space where you can talk about your experiences and validate the experiences of others. Safe spaces are places where you can escape scrutiny and surround yourself with others like you. It's a place where you can authentically be you without code-switching (which is adjusting your language, tone, style of dress, or some other marker of a marginalized identity to fit in with the majority). You're looking for someplace you can shed your professional veneer and just be personal. A place where you don't have to cover up your true emotions or explain why it's not all right to compare a Black person to a lump of coal or joke about someone's pronouns.

Safe spaces can take on plenty of different forms. You might have a forward-thinking job that encourages employee resource groups for Hispanic Americans or the LGBTQ community. They can create safe spaces where you can talk about workplace micro- and macroaggressions, like a supervisor who asked to touch your hair. There are even safe spaces within safe spaces. For example, Alcoholics Anonymous and Narcotics Anonymous meetings create protected environments for talking about addiction. But even within these groups there are smaller groups for African Americans in recovery for alcoholism and for people who are Gay & Sober.

I also encourage my patients to google—in very specific terms—what they're going through to find local support groups, online meetings, closed Facebook groups, anonymous venting Reddit threads, and more. You might try "Jamaican immigrants who just lost a baby online support," "support resources for adolescent female athletes near me," or "Asian people that struggle with alcoholism in Jacksonville, Florida." There are so many small, hidden resources on the internet that you might never find by word of mouth alone.

Interacting with a group might be the last thing you want to do after a long day of micro- or macroaggressions from family you had to spend the holidays with, neighbors you run into coming in and out of your home, or coworkers you've been around all day. Your safe space can be just one other person: a single coworker with whom you have a shared experience, a best friend who always listens, a therapist who gets it.

There's no right or wrong way to start your "safe space" conversation. If you show up for a group meeting, there will probably be ground rules. If your safe space is smaller, you might send a Slack to a safe space coworker after an awkward meeting that says, "Girl, can we duck out for lunch so I can talk to you about what just happened?" Or you might text a friend a quick "Got a minute? I need to vent." Or email your therapist and let her know something happened that you really need to talk about in your next session. Or now. It's all right and even important to specifically ask for what you want: the need to get

HOW WEATHERING ANY STORM CAN WITHER YOUR HEALTH

something off your chest. The validation that what happened was not okay. The desire to express to someone exactly how angry, sad, frustrated, confused, exhausted that experience made you feel.

Some days you'll be the person seeking the shelter in a discrimination storm. Other days you'll be the person that someone is coming to—and there are powerful ways in which you can show up for that person. When someone comes to you needing safe space:

Thank them for doing so. Reassure them that their self-care outreach was well received. Thank them for coming to speak with you.

Be fully present with them. It's going to be tempting to guess how the story ends or jump in and talk about the exact same time something like this happened to you. Don't. This isn't the Adversity Olympics. It's an opportunity to help someone heal by being a good listener and a great advocate. Also, you might find yourself starting to get angry or upset or matching their energy. Try to stay calm and focused on what they're going through. Your number one goal in this moment is validation. That can be a knowing glance, a slow nod, a sad shake of your head, or figurative clutching of the pearls. It could sound as simple as "Oh no!" or "I get it" or "I'm so sorry that happened."

Ask open-ended questions. Avoid questions that can be answered with a yes or no. That way you don't introduce your own bias into what someone is sharing, and you enable them to have more space to think about what happened. For example, you wouldn't ask: "Sounds like you have a bad relationship with this neighbor, huh?" Instead, you'd say: "How would you describe your relationship with this lady?"

Ask them what they want. You might find yourself just dying to give some advice. "Man, what you need to do is . . ." or "You know what you should tell her?" Don't. Ask the person who has come to you what they need. They may have just wanted to get it off their chest. They might be looking to de-escalate the situation. You won't know until you ask them what they need in that moment.

Avoid re-traumatizing them. No one's thinking of the perfect quip when they get broadsided by discrimination and racism. So, when they share what happened to them, avoid making them feel bad about not having the perfect response by saying something like, "If that was me, I would've told them off." or "That would never happen in my family and if it did, I'd put that person to shame."

Be respectful of their space. Physical touch isn't for everyone. Be mindful of your friend's personal space. After a trauma, you might catch a person in freeze mode, but they could also be in fight-or-flight and not quite up for a reach out and touch moment. Whether you want to put your hand on top of theirs or go for a full-body hug that you resolve to be the last person to pull away from, just ask. I'm a hugger so I've always been in the habit of just saying, "Would it be all right to give you a hug?" People appreciate it and will usually tell you the truth.

We all make mistakes. And there's a chance that you'll find yourself in a situation where you've said or done something that was received as a microaggression by someone else. If they approach you, again, thank them for coming to you to let you know what you've done wrong. If you need to approach them:

Own your errant ways. You could say, "I was thinking about the meeting we were in the other day. I realize I might have said something or done something that didn't land well with you. That wasn't my intent."

HOW WEATHERING ANY STORM CAN WITHER YOUR HEALTH

Show your work. Make the other person aware that your intent is to take the burden of rectifying the situation off of them and onto you. You can say, "I wouldn't want you to have to be the one to come to me about this incident. I take it as my responsibility to create the space for you to be able to tell me if what I said didn't land well."

End on a positive. Reiterate that you're glad they allowed you to have the conversation and that you want to keep this type of communication open going forward.

Finally, you may be on the sidelines watching the macroaggression take place. Instead of being an innocent bystander who shakes their head and moves on, you can be an active upstander and help to heal the situation. It's up to you whether you want to approach the injured party or the macroaggressor. Either way, here's what you might say:

Reassure the offended individual. "Wow, that comment from the meeting really bothered me. If it landed the same way with you, I wanted to acknowledge that." Sometimes it's clear that the offender meant to offend. But if you believe it could've been a mistake, you could say something like, "I assume that person who offended you has good intent and wouldn't want to intentionally hurt your feelings. I'd like to encourage them to speak with you about what they said. Is that all right?"

Give the offender a heads-up. "It didn't impact me directly, but what you said at the meeting pinged my radar. Here are some reasons why it would be considered offensive by other people who were in the room. I think you might want to go speak with [insert name] and let them know that your intention wasn't to offend."

Un-Addicted: Your Acquired Psychological Risk

You've had some time to look at the negative consequences of discrimination in a whole new way. Discrimination works on a psychological and biological level to impact longevity, wellness, resilience, and more. I know it's a lot, so I've narrowed things down. These are the concepts I hope you'll focus on.

Key Takeaways

» **Weathering wears down your ability to experience good health.**
Weathering is the process through which racism, discrimination, and marginalization remove stable blocks (or pillars of health and wellness) from a structure. Remove too much stability and eventually that structure (or person) will collapse.

» **Your overall health and risk of addiction are tied to your experience with discrimination and adversity.**
You can't treat substance use disorders without addressing the impact of choiceless states (e.g., race and gender). In terms of addiction, they impact your risk, your treatment in recovery, and the legal consequences you may experience.

» **A sense of belonging can be a shield or a scepter in the face of discrimination.**
Racism and discrimination are modern-day equivalents of exiling individuals from the pack. Having a group or even

just one other person that understands you can be protective against the impact of racism and discrimination. Everyone needs a safe space to simply be themself.

Your Homework

» **Do a deep dive on your own experience with discrimination.**
Journal about a time when an experience with racism, discrimination, or marginalization impacted your mood or even caused you to turn to substance use. Think about the thoughts and feelings you had in that moment. How long did it take you to recover from that experience? The goal is to recognize how deeply these experiences affect our thoughts and emotions.

» **Seek to understand someone else's experience.**
Choose a loved one or even a stranger and consider how their experiences with racism, discrimination, or marginalization may impact their mood or drive substance use. Considering the invisible battles that people around us are fighting builds compassion and understanding.

» **Put your pulse to the test.**
Take your pulse to determine your resting heart rate (number of beats per minute) while you're calm. Now do the same test after thinking about an experience with racism, discrimination, or marginalization that you've experienced. You'll likely notice your heart rate increase by ten to fifteen beats, showing you the link between choiceless states and health.

⟫ Have more safe space conversations.

Expressing yourself takes practice. So does finding the right words when someone else needs to talk to you. Seek out opportunities to flex those muscles by also considering talking to someone when your first reaction to a frustrating situation is the impulse to vent on social media or pull away from loved ones. Pay attention to the times when a friend or colleague is upset and you're at a loss for words—use that as an opportunity to offer to listen. You'll improve your ability to get and give the support you need.

CHAPTER SIX
Scrolling Toward Addiction
From social media to national holidays– the cultures and environments that encourage risky substance use

In the 2010s, smoking was making a comeback—and it had never looked sexier. As the popularity of cigarettes was taking some of its final breaths, a new nicotine delivery system was on the rise: vaping. Electronic cigarettes didn't just bill themselves as a safer and less offensive alternative to smoking. One company built an entire #LightsCameraVapor mystique around the newest way to inhale. On social media, swirling wisps of white vapor escaped the open mouths of anyone you could imagine: scantily clad young models who looked like they were having the time of their life; handsome influencers who were so cool they could barely make eye contact with you in their posts; regular people who wanted in on the latest new trend. At a launch party in June 2015, electronic cigarette company Juul tweeted out a photo showing a group of five extremely hip-looking girls in midi dresses and black leather with vape pens and party cups in their hands. The tweet read: "Having way too much fun at the #JUUL launch party."

UN-ADDICTION

Culturally, puffing on a cigarette used to make you look cool, mysterious, interesting, and even sexy. Now, e-cigarettes were taking over that narrative. But the ads had come a long way from Virginia Slims days. Instead of the rugged, older Marlboro man, you saw a younger, hipper guy who could pass for a high schooler. Young models were likely a strategy to not only capture an older demographic obsessed with youth, but also get interest from a younger one, including teenagers and younger kids. Every successful business always needs to think about new customer acquisitions.

In 2014, nearly 70 percent of middle and high school–aged children were exposed to e-cigarette ads whether they were online, in retail stores, in magazines or newspapers, on television or in movies. Plus, those whiffs of smoke can taste like Pineapple Peach Mango, Vanilla Custard, and Melontini to appeal to adults or Crunch Berry, Grape Slush, and Hard Candy, flavors that would undoubtedly appeal to young kids. The flavors were a game-changer. In fact, one study of eleven- to sixteen-year-old nonsmokers showed that ads for flavored e-cigarettes (compared to those without flavor) increased interest in buying and trying e-cigarettes. What e-cigarette companies were selling, kids were buying.

By 2018, Juul, which held the vast majority of the e-cigarette market, was on track to become a billion-dollar company. They had increased their revenue 300 percent from the previous year mostly by throwing their efforts into marketing on social media. Which makes it shocking that they decided to shut down their Instagram and Facebook accounts the exact same year. Why would they lean away from the marketing techniques that were helping them make hundreds of millions of dollars? Because the marketing was working too well. Runaway train well. It wasn't only adult consumers who were paying attention to Juul on social media. Researchers were taking notice as well. Their studies showed that exposure to social media posts about e-cigarettes was tied to a greater risk for e-cigarette use among adolescents—which weren't supposed to be a nicotine company's demographic.

One study showed that four out of five students overestimated how much their peers were vaping. The risk of that belief was that it might just lead to them vaping even more. Consenting adults was one thing. But young adults under eighteen scrolling through their feed and getting hooked? That was something entirely different. Even the Food and Drug Administration took note and got involved.

When We Talk About Culture, What Do We Mean?

Like biology and psychology, culture is a significant source of our risk of developing addiction. And how does it relate to substance use? Culture is the collection of social customs that become ingrained in our everyday existence. On a macro level, it's the holidays and customs that make up the fabric of American life. It's a long-held national Thanksgiving Day tradition of eating so much we can barely roll ourselves away from the dining table and onto the couch. Or that every Cinco de Mayo, there's an expectation of getting so drunk that you might not make it to work on time the next day. It's an environment that has us all buying chocolate for Valentine's Day and judging million-dollar commercials while dipping chips in guac with our best friends on Super Bowl

UN-ADDICTION

Sunday. It's a society that tells us it's cool to spike our water with booze because hard seltzer is delicious. And, by the way, buying in bulk is better because supersize matters! It's a social agreement that at twenty-one years of age, it's okay (maybe even expected) for you to get so drunk that you can't even look at vodka again for another twenty-one years.

On a micro level, it's the things you might take for granted in your family, like celebrating the anniversary of a family member's passing so you never forget them or taking a family photo every year so that you can see how everyone has changed over the decades. It may be the fact that everyone in your family (like my extended family) gathers around to do shots on holidays—even filling shot glasses for the kids in the family with Sprite or Kool-Aid so they can join in the indoctrination. It's the way some social circles accept getting hazed to pledge a fraternity while others are devoted to volunteerism.

Culture is aesthetics and the way that language is used. It's the reason that people at a jazz club look and sound different than those at an Afropunk festival. It's the song lyrics that are laced with references to marijuana, alcohol, smoking, cocaine, and more. The words we're singing along to are sending powerful messages across all genres. In fact, some research shows that country music songs have the highest reference to drug use. All those songs about cold beer and warm tears add up to more than you'd expect.

This culture is in the media that we consume—from the thirty-second advertisements and commercials that tell us what's sexy, to the social media posts that tell us how to relax, to the television shows we get invested in. It's the way we accept watching mom Georgia, on *Ginny & Georgia*, walk into a bar and have the owner pour her a glass of exactly what she wants without her having to say anything. Or how we don't question Olivia Pope downing a glass of Bordeaux as her coping mechanism after "handling" a *Scandal*. It's the way we barely notice that Bow on *Black-ish* is rarely seen at home without a glass of wine in her hand. Culture is what makes us swoon a bit when an actor we love leans over and lights the cigarette of his love interest on-screen. It makes us wish we were in on the fun when we see a group of women out on a girls' night drinking or a circle of friends at a club dropping Ecstasy.

There's a culture around your profession. Whether used as a social lubricant at networking events or a way to let off steam after an endless day of meetings, what you do for a living could be inextricably tied to substance use.

I once had a musician client whose livelihood was built around playing gigs in bars: small venues filled with people asking the bartender for one more drink or heading into a back room to do illicit drugs. If your work culture is bandmates and fellow artists who use and who might trigger cravings in you to use substances, imagine how difficult it might be to get and stay sober. I have a lot of artists who tell me they feel less creative when they're not using. That *not* using drugs inhibits the vibrancy or beauty of the paintings, music, book, sculpture, or script that they bring to the world. That using allows them to access the part of their brain that creates and is actually part of their self-identity, joy, and sense of purpose as well. I have to understand that asking them to change people, places, and things may very well feel like asking them to lose everything they know and love about themselves.

Culture is also your politics, religion, and the laws by which you abide. The fact that we can buy alcohol that is regulated by a government entity makes us believe it is safe, maybe unlike buying moonshine from the lady in the backwoods. Getting a prescription for opioids or marijuana from a doctor may make me feel better than going to a dispensary out of state or even a drug dealer because the FDA has endorsed it, even though it has the potential to be equally dangerous. One phrase that has always driven me crazy is: "It's just marijuana." That language and the legalization of this drug are also part of our culture. They make it sound like there is nothing dangerous about marijuana, or that nothing negative could come from using it. Neither is true.

Growing up, my father was an avid marijuana smoker. That's part of my ACEs and my inherited environment right there. The smell of marijuana turned my stomach. The secondhand smoke burned my eyes and made me cough. But this was in the '70s when marijuana use was at an all-time high. Think anti-war revolutionaries, political activists, and hippies all blazing up as part of the "anti-culture." My dad and his friends, while high, seemed useless to me. They pontificated on lofty ideas that, in my mind, were . . . well, dumb. I saw my parents having conflict about marijuana. "Reefer," as my dad called it, was frequently at the center of their arguments. By third grade, I had decided marijuana was an awful drug that I would never try. Back then, I didn't know what I know now as an addiction psychiatrist. What I was experiencing was a father with post-traumatic stress disorder from combat in Vietnam who was attempting to medicate away his symptoms and developing a cannabis use disorder in the process.

Fast-forward to my freshman year of college, and there I was, trying marijuana. My environment had changed, and along with it came the culture of college. My people, places, and things had changed. Why I decided to smoke that night, I can't be entirely sure, but I would bet it had to do with the supercute guy who oozed edgy New Yorker vibes and lived in an off-campus apartment. Even at that point in my life, trying to impress wasn't my style, but there was something about him. We smoked, and I choked. I immediately became nauseous, and my eyes started to burn. I thought to myself, annoyed, "You knew better." But then, something happened—and I'm not kidding about this part. I could see without my glasses. I went room to room in the apartment exclaiming to anyone who would listen: "I can see! I can see! With no glasses! I can see!"

Everyone told me after the fact that it was hilarious. But I had experienced something that was not so funny. While yes, I had been amazed that I really could see without my glasses, I also felt my self-control slipping as the intoxication set in. I heard myself pontificating. Simultaneously, I hated it, but at the same time felt a compulsion to smoke even more to intensify it. Even while still high, I envisioned myself as my marijuana-addicted father from my younger years. I knew I would never smoke again. And I didn't.

A few years later, I graduated from Howard and went to Penn Medicine, where, as described earlier in the book, I shocked everyone, myself included, by deciding to become an addiction psychiatrist. Once I finished psychiatric training at Emory University in Atlanta, I accepted a job as staff psychiatrist, splitting my time between the mental health clinic, where I practiced harm reduction, and the addiction clinic, where I was the psychiatrist for a complete abstinence-based program. I took my disdain for marijuana with me.

As I began practicing in the addiction clinic, I noticed marijuana was one of the more frequent substances that my patients had difficulty quitting. Their drug screens would turn negative for cocaine (the most common drug being used in the clinic at that time), but marijuana use persisted. In the mental health clinic, the connection between heavy marijuana use and schizophrenia in my young Black male patients was undeniable. In the addiction clinic, I spent each day trying to convince my patients that the legal risks of marijuana outweighed the benefits. In the mental health clinic, I implored my patients to stop smoking with hopes that doing so would lessen their psychotic symptoms. Still, it didn't take long for my enthusiasm for anti-marijuana activism to begin waning.

I saw mothers lose custody of their children because of marijuana. I saw fathers go to jail because of marijuana. I saw young adult children get kicked out of their parents' homes because of marijuana. What I didn't see was stealing, or violent crimes, or overdose deaths because of marijuana. I couldn't help asking the question: Why had the legal consequences of marijuana far outpaced the physiological consequences? The answer is criminalization of drug use and addiction. Shortly after asking myself that question, as an abstinence-based addiction psychiatrist, I became a proponent of legalizing marijuana. Fifteen years later, that cultural change is happening right now before our eyes. Recreational marijuana use is being legalized in multiple states and use is at a thirty-year all-time high.

Now remember, I started this whole story with "just because it's legal doesn't mean it's safe." Alcohol and cigarettes account for more than 600,000 deaths each year in the U.S. Likewise, just because I support the legalization of marijuana doesn't mean it is without risks. Nearly three in ten people who use marijuana regularly meet the diagnostic criteria for marijuana use disorder, and I have certainly taken care of patients who have become addicted to marijuana and nearly lost their family, their sense of self, and their livelihood as a result. I already mentioned the young men I took care of whose marijuana use was worsening their psychosis. And it's a well-documented medical fact that those young people who start using marijuana before the age of fourteen have increased risk for difficulties with mental health, problem-solving, memory, learning, and maintaining attention.

For this reason, I educate my kids on their inherited biological risk factor for addiction and recommend they don't try it. But understanding that marijuana smoking, vaping, and edibles are quickly becoming a common part of high school culture, if they do try it, I've shared with them the red flags that might indicate they are losing control of their use. I counsel my adult patients with addiction, depression, asthma or other lung diseases, anxiety, or symptoms of ADHD to stop using marijuana, or as a harm reduction strategy, to switch from smoking to vaping to edibles, to decrease the negative impact of marijuana on their other symptoms.

Understanding my own risk, I continue to say "No thank you" when my friends offer edibles or a bong while we're on ski trips in Colorado. And I'll tell you, those conversations used to be a lot easier to have before the culture changed to a full-on embrace of recreational marijuana use. But the culture around a substance doesn't always change to make things harder for abstainers. Sometimes it changes in a way that makes it easier to just say "No thank you." That's exactly what happened when one large company started a cultural revolution of its own that had a bigger impact than any of us could've expected.

When a Goliath Went Up Against a Goliath

Two billion dollars was on the line. The year was 2013 and Larry J. Merlo, CEO and president of the company that was about to let those two billion dollars slip between its fingers, was trying to figure out what to do. Would his company, CVS Health, continue to sell tobacco products while claiming to care about the health of Americans? They would lose two billion in sales if they stopped. Or would CVS Health clear its shelves of one of the largest threats to American public health in history? Worldwide, tobacco kills seven million people every single year and in the United States it takes the lives of nearly a half million annually. It was one of those classic questions of people versus profit. Walking the walk and talking the talk. But it was also a question of acquired environmental risk factors for addiction. How had we gotten to a place where it was culturally acceptable to pick up your asthma medication from the same place you grabbed a pack of Marlboros?

As Merlo was steering the company to have a bigger health impact on a local level, the predicament made him wonder: Was tobacco going to be a financial enabler or a hypocritical barrier to CVS Health's growth? Would they rebrand and emerge with a bigger purpose? Or try to keep explaining why an addiction-causing, cancer-causing product was still sold behind the counter? It wasn't only his decision to make, though. So, Merlo took that question to the board of directors.

Consumer Value Stores, now known as CVS, has come a long way since its humble beginnings as a health and beauty supply store in Lowell, Massachusetts, in 1963. Only a few years after it opened, it started placing pharmacies within its stores. Then healthcare clinics.

SCROLLING TOWARD ADDICTION

In just a few decades of rapid growth and acquisition, it became one of the biggest drugstore chains in the United States. Today, roughly 70 percent of the United States lives within three miles of a CVS. CVS and all it stands for and sells is reflective of American culture. The corporation's influence on communities throughout the country cannot be overstated.

But what exactly is the responsibility of a store to the community it serves and the environments where it exists? In 2013, CVS Health was a chain with a bit of an existential crisis trying to answer the question of how much they wanted to impact the health of those communities. They were also on the heels of acquiring Aetna, a health insurance company, in a $69 billion deal. So perhaps it was no wonder that the board decided quickly about the tobacco situation. In fact, it only took a half hour. They would stop selling tobacco products in their stores because it was the right thing for a healthcare company to do.

By September 3, 2014, cigarettes, chewing tobacco, and other tobacco products were cleared from CVS Health's shelves. CVS Health became the first pharmacy chain to stop selling tobacco products in the U.S. That day, Merlo was front and center on the New York Stock Exchange balcony with more than a dozen colleagues as they rang the opening bell. Changing the country on a random Wednesday. Not a bad day's work. Despite the announcement that they were dropping products that brought in two billion annually, CVS Health's stock didn't tank. It rose. Steadily. For the next year.

Image matters. But what CVS Health was also trying to do was to make an impact on the environments it inhabited. They wanted to have a local effect on healthcare access and meet people where they were with their health goals. It worked. Cigarette sales dropped in areas where CVS had a significant presence. Research found that 95 million fewer packs of cigarettes were sold across the country in the first year that CVS Health made this change. The average smoker in markets where CVS had a significant presence purchased five fewer packs of cigarettes that year. CVS found that people who exclusively bought their cigarettes from CVS were about 38 percent more likely to stop buying cigarettes altogether once the store stopped selling them. Here was proof that limiting access to cigarettes (basically changing the environment and culture around a substance) could reduce tobacco use.

I tell you this story to highlight another massive impact that the political culture we commit to has on our health. We're all used to government making these kinds of decisions about our culture and environment. By 1920, the entire country had delved into a decade of prohibition. Prohibition, enforced by the Eighteenth Amendment to the Constitution, banned the manufacture, transportation, and sale of intoxicating liquors. The hope was to improve public health and safety, strengthen families, save grain for food during World War I, and more. In 1995, California became the first state to ban smoking in every workplace and indoor public space. It completely changed the experience of what we think of today as going to a restaurant or a club—which is still going strong today. We have laws that prevent people from being able to buy alcohol until they turn twenty-one and stop companies from advertising cigarettes—all in the interest of trying to reduce acquired environmental factors that increase the risk of addiction.

What I really want to drive home with the CVS story is what can happen when the environment and culture you're born into changes—through no effort of your own—to reduce your risk and/or support your sobriety. And it isn't just brought on by billion-dollar corporations. It could be brought on by a new school you attend, a new job culture, a new religion you choose, a new family you marry into, a new city you move to.

Understanding the Sneaky, Subversive Impact of Culture

Resisting the culture of an addiction—by not pledging a certain fraternity at your college so you can avoid partying or binge drinking on your twenty-first birthday—can be extremely difficult. Culture infiltrates our lives every single day without us realizing it. But researchers realize it. Studies have shown that the less Latinx immigrants who come to this country acculturate, the less risk they have for susceptibility to addiction. Another study of more than 3,500 Asian Americans showed that those who were born in the U.S. had the highest heavy-drinking levels, followed by longtime-resident Asian immigrants, and then recent-resident immigrants. Other factors besides how long the individuals had been in the States were also at play, but the importance of time spent in our supersized, buying-in-bulk, instant gratification, fix-it-with-a-pill, drink-away-your-sorrows American culture is fairly undeniable.

Cultural influences are extremely difficult to overcome—even when we're aware of their impact. Consciously going against the grain can be exhausting. I remember listening to the producer of a local radio show talk about a friend who started drinking heavily in college. He decided he wanted to cut back but needed some help. The producer immediately jumped in to help. "We will figure out a way to have you drink less," she assured him. She crowdsourced ideas that worked for other people. Did research online. Talked to experts. And then went back to him with a plan that included her detoxing with him. Or did it? "Do I really want to give up liquor?" she had to ask herself. Was she really ready not to go to bars to hang out with her friends? Was she willing not to unwind at the end of a long day with a glass of wine? Or not to get excited about the latest new cocktail that everyone was buzzing about?

In the end they made a plan that both of them could manage. Instead of traditional bars, they went to zero-proof bars where the sober drinks taste as great as the ones with alcohol in them. That cultural impact is massive. You can still go to a lounge. You can modify your place, tweak your things, and still keep your people.

It may not seem like a big deal reading about it. So how about you give it a try? Just for one day—or maybe two so you can feel the impact on a weekday and a weekend. I'm going to challenge you to notice how many times any sort of substance appears in your life. Pick one. It could be tequila or cigarettes. Chocolate or potato chips. Focus on one item and notice every single time that one of your senses is called to buy or consume it. How often are you seeing TV commercials or written advertisements for that substance? How often do you walk down the street and smell it or see people consuming it? How often do you see a friend using it or talking about it? How much space in your local stores is devoted to selling it? Get tuned in to how much that substance is woven into the fabric of society and into the culture that you're immersed in. It's probably in the neighborhood of hundreds or even thousands of times a day that some substance is put in front of your face to tantalize you to consume it. Now take a step back and realize that you just did an experiment for a day. Imagine if every single day of your life were like that because you were working on maintaining your goal of complete abstinence or controlled use of that substance. Remember, the dopamine signal that's driving you back to that substance is fierce: your environment and your biology are on one side of the tug-of-war rope and you're on the other.

It's not possible to put yourself in a bubble to avoid the impact of drug culture. But you can do things to protect yourself. One of those things is taking a short quiz that goes a long way to helping you and your healthcare professionals understand the culture and environment in which you currently live.

The Cultural Impact Questionnaire

I know healthcare providers often get a (sometimes well-deserved) bad rap. But truth is, most of us really do care and we really do want what's best for you. This is why we make our best effort to meet our patients where they are. To really do so, we have to take your cultural experiences and how they are affecting your health into consideration. That's what I mean when I reference culturally relevant care. Now, because we are human, and subject to all the implicit biases just like anyone else, of course I'm going to recommend a standardized tool to help us have this conversation—the Cultural Formulation Interview.

Created by the American Psychiatric Association (APA), the questionnaire is meant to help clinicians improve their culturally relevant care for all types of mental health concerns: depression, anxiety, eating disorders, substance use disorders, and more. It gives healthcare providers insight into how you make decisions and offers us a better understanding about you and the environment in which you exist.

I'm including an abbreviated version of the questionnaire that I've adapted to focus on substance use and substance use disorders. You've heard me say this before to manage expectations and it remains true: Not every doctor is going to ask you these cultural questions—and they almost certainly won't ask you these questions in relation to substance use disorders. Regardless of what your provider does, you can take the quiz yourself to better understand how your behaviors may be influencing your health risk and to share the results.

For each question, think about and write down an answer before delving into the reasoning behind the question that follows in the text. It's a clinical survey meant for professionals, so I want you to include your gut reaction or initial response to each question and then I will break down what your healthcare provider is looking for in your answers.

Cultural Formulation Interview

1. For you, what are the most important aspects of your identity and your upbringing?

What I love about this question is that it enables your healthcare provider to take culturally relevant care to the next level. For example, just because I meet with another Black woman who is a patient doesn't mean that we have the same identity. She might consider being a woman the biggest part of her identity while I might consider being

Black the most important aspect of mine. This question lets your healthcare provider get to the heart of who you are, from your perspective, regardless of how you appear to their eyes.

When you're thinking of your answers to the question of identity, it makes sense to lean into the REGaLS (Race, Ethnicity, Gender Identity, Language, Sexuality) that I shared in the previous chapter. Maybe your identity is being bisexual. Or Latinx. REGaLS are a great place to start, but you should venture beyond them as well. Your identity could also be tied to the role you play as a mother, as an artist, or as an environmentalist. Your family has a culture that is probably different from other families. That's tied to your identity, too. The school you went to has a culture. Your profession has a culture. Even the fact that you're in recovery could be part of your identity. Traditional abstinence-based programs tell their clients that the most important aspect of their identity is as a recovering addict—their words, not mine! But you may not want addiction (or any other illness) to be the defining part of your identity, let alone the only identity that others recognize. That's important for your healthcare provider to know.

When you're considering your upbringing, think about the most important aspects of your upbringing that made you the person you are today. You might come up with ideas about your economic status, whether your parents were divorced, or whether you're a down-home country girl or a concrete-jungle-loving city guy.

2. Are there any aspects of your background or identity that make a difference to your risk of developing a substance use disorder?

This question will help your healthcare practitioner identify what parts of your identity could increase your risk or make your recovery more difficult. In Irish culture, for example, it's often a badge of honor to be able to outdrink everybody else and binge drinking is considered the norm. I've taken care of people with Irish backgrounds and it's clear that their upbringing exposed them to a culture around alcohol that encouraged use and made it harder to stop drinking. Trying to be abstinent from alcohol often becomes a situation in which my Irish patients have to choose—stop drinking or be with their family. As you can imagine, that can be an excruciating decision to be faced with.

One of my patients told me about an upcoming wedding and how stressed she was to attend. Something that should be pure happiness was joyless to think about because she knew what would happen as soon as she arrived at the reception. It was an impossible situation: She wanted to go to the wedding because it's a beautiful milestone, but she wanted to RSVP no because it was putting her sobriety at risk. She ended up attending, but white-knuckled it in the corner for the entire reception. She didn't drink, but it also didn't feel like a success. Other guests kept saying things like, "Why are you sitting over there by yourself?" and "You didn't even join the party." They weren't trying to be mean. They honestly didn't understand the struggle. But when you share these cultural hurdles with your healthcare provider, I hope they will not only understand, but also help you make a plan to address them—or connect you to a professional who can.

3. Are there any aspects of your background or identity that are causing other concerns or difficulties for you?

This question is all about the different ways that society makes life, health, and recovery difficult for people based on their background or identity. It's about how we can be made to feel like an outsider even when we are just being ourselves. Maybe it's the fact that you are a person with a disability and being blind, deaf, or navigating the world in a wheelchair makes it harder to access culturally relevant care. Perhaps you're a gay woman and it's difficult to find a gynecologist who understands your sexual life. You might even be seeking care for obesity and experiencing discrimination from the provider you've entrusted to help.

4. Sometimes people have various ways of dealing with problems like a substance use disorder. What have you done on your own to cope with your substance use disorder?

Simply put, this question is asking: "Before you got to me, what did you try?" I have multiple patients who went from being addicted to pain pills (like OxyContin or Vicodin) to being addicted to kratom, an unregulated, opioid-like substance that people think is natural. They feel better using a supplement than coming to get a prescription from a doctor. When a patient responds to these questions by telling me about everything they've tried under the sun (herbs, supplements, self-help books, church, picking up a new hobby), that tells me that I need to listen carefully and understand what it is about coming to me, a doctor, that feels so unsafe that it has to be saved as a last resort. In this type of situation, I know that it's even more important than usual to work to create a safe environment and have transparent conversations. This will help me avoid re-creating a healthcare experience that might make it harder for you to reach your goals.

5. Often, people look for help from many different sources, including different kinds of doctors, helpers, or healers. In the past, what kinds of treatment, help, advice, or healing have you sought for your substance use disorder? What types of help or treatment were most useful? Not useful?

This question is about other practitioners that you went to. Maybe you decided to give acupuncture or Chinese medicine a try. You may have gone to see a cognitive behavioral therapist. Or perhaps you went to a Reiki healer in your community. Or you decided to visit a medical intuitive who said they could solve your problem for you. Maybe you spent an afternoon in Barnes & Noble looking at personal development books. All of this helps me understand what type of practitioners you feel comfortable with—and if possible, we will want to incorporate those practitioners in your care plan.

6. Has anything prevented you from getting the help you need?

So many things can prevent us from asking for help or getting the help that we need: stigma, not having a single sick day from your job, family culture that says to pull yourself up by your bootstraps, our religious beliefs. I once had a Muslim client who had an addiction to heroin. It all started with the pressures of immigrating to the United States from another country right after graduating high school. He was under a tremendous amount of pressure to succeed in college, which led to him taking pills to decrease his anxiety and homesickness. Eventually his pill use turned into heroin use that he could no longer control.

While many people lean on their faith or religion for strength during hard times, religious beliefs can also sometimes be a barrier to getting help. In this patient's case, being Muslim meant that alcohol and other drug use was strictly prohibited. Believing that he had betrayed his religious beliefs made it extremely difficult for him to seek help. When he did seek help, his religious beliefs meant that he could not be alone in a room with a female doctor or therapist. The field of medicine is heavy with men. But psychiatry and psychotherapy are mostly women. We didn't have any male therapists in our practice at the time, but asking this question gave us the opportunity to understand that to adequately serve this patient's needs, we had to find one.

7. Are there other kinds of help that your family, friends, or other people have suggested would be helpful for you now?

This question tells me three important things. First, it reveals whether you have a support circle that you feel you can lean on. Second, it lets me know if your circle is concerned about you. Finally, if they did raise concerns, it tells me whether they were able to raise their concerns in a compassionate and helpful way, and if you were able to receive their concerns as being driven by good intent. Your support system can have the best of intentions but still not approach you in an effective way.

Or, your support system might approach you in an effective way, and you still may not be open to receive the feedback they are sharing. All of it is information that helps me understand what type of support might be helpful for you and for your support system. But what about the times when your support system doesn't have the best of intentions? They may even be pressuring you to use when you're trying to make a different decision. Let's talk about what to do if you find yourself in that situation.

How to Handle Peer Pressure Even When You're an Adult

We tend to think of peer pressure as being confined to our teenage years, but the truth is, no matter how old (or young at heart) we are, most of us have a ferocious need to be a part of the pack. Research shows that it's actually baked into how we've evolved as humans. We've developed into beings who are overly influenced by those around us.

Herd mentality is neurobiologically hardwired into our brains. That animal instinct has a lot going for it. The same way that herds of animals move together knowing there is safety in numbers and that they decrease their chances of getting picked off by a predator, humans do the same thing. We do it on a survival level: Think about the ways that we mostly cluster together in urban areas rather than living isolated by ourselves. Think about the last time you watched video of an event where someone heard a gunshot, and a group of people all ran in the same direction away from it. We also do it on a superficial level. Ever felt pressured into buying crypto instead of stocks? Or had the

SCROLLING TOWARD ADDICTION

urge to quit shaving or let someone pour a bucket of ice over your head for the sake of a social media challenge everyone else was doing?

Navigating social situations where you are the only one using an Android phone in a sea of iPhones can feel like you're practically self-exiling—or putting yourself at risk for getting kicked out of the pack. It can also simply leave you at a loss for words during times you really need those words! It's to graciously accept when a host automatically places a glass of champagne in your hand on New Year's Eve. It's to puff puff pass when someone hands you a joint. While the instinct to follow the crowd is built into our brain, so is the need for nurturing. Remember when I told you about how nurturing is one of our primal needs? Pretty hard to feel that when you're being exiled from the pack for rejecting the accepted culture. "What do you mean you haven't seen *The Wire*?" "How is it possible that you've never had an Impossible Burger?"

As a society, we're constantly evolving. We've learned how to stop assuming someone's gender identity and accept the pronouns they choose as indicated in their email signature or Zoom call description. We've recognized the need to reinforce that no means no at any point of the night and have leaned into that messaging in sex education classes, movies, and in the media. If we can shift these types of behaviors, no doubt we can rethink how we offer substances to people, how we accept a polite decline, and how we confidently voice a hard pass. We can decide to stop giving people a hard time if they don't want to get smashed at the bachelorette party. We can make a conscious choice to reconsider whether smoking actually makes that character on television look cooler, smarter, or sexier. We can choose not to put the weed dispensary on the getaway trip itinerary even though we will be in Colorado.

I absolutely believe that we can retrain, reprogram, and recondition our minds to think more broadly, behave more compassionately, and speak more confidently in environments where we may feel culturally pressured to use a substance. And I'll take it one step further. Not only do I believe it, but I also don't think it has to be hard. I know because the process I'm about to teach you is exactly what I work on with my patients. It can work for you if you're at high risk of developing a substance use disorder, and it can also work for you when you're simply coming up against cultural pressures around substance use that you don't want to succumb to.

In recovery, we help patients to:

- **Recognize what triggers them to want to use a substance.**
- **Avoid those triggers.**
- **Plan for what to do when they can't sidestep a situation.**

So, if you know having a dinner meeting with your boss will mean cognac and cigars, perhaps you try to take him to lunch instead. And if you absolutely must meet over dinner, you arrive early and make sure the waiter knows you're not drinking and offers you alternatives.

The same strategies apply even if you are not in recovery. The goal is to recognize the situations where you could be pressured into using. Then you want to avoid those situations and come up with a plan for when you're stuck in them. When it comes to recognizing situations, there are probably some recurring events that immediately come to mind. Maybe you know those Sunday brunches with your girlfriends always bring some big announcements (engagements, pregnancies, divorces) and an endless flow of drinks (Bellinis, Bloody Marys, mimosas) that you're not interested in. *You don't need the calories, don't want that exhausted feeling that comes later, can't afford the bill, or have zero interest in a hangover.* All valid reasons but none of them make it easier to be the only person sipping club soda and laughing at a reasonable volume at the table. Maybe your buddies have been talking about a vacation in Peru where everyone can sit in a yurt with a shaman and do ayahuasca under the stars. You're not interested in finding yourself through a full-blown mystical experience, but that doesn't make it any easier to swallow the idea of sitting at the hotel by yourself for half a day.

These are all situations that require planning in the first place, so you can plan to avoid temptations like smoking marijuana just because you're in Amsterdam. And, by the way, these avoidance plans don't mean that you have to skip out on these experiences altogether. You can avoid undesired outcomes by having a plan for what to do when you find yourself in a less than optimal situation. You can still go to brunch, but have a conversation with your circle beforehand about doing a dry January or having plans after brunch that you need to be sober for. You can make the Peru trip with your buddies but plan a daytrip to entertain yourself while they're out in that tent—and you might even make them jealous with the pics you capture.

Few things make deviating from the "norm" easier than having an ally. Pick one person who'll be attending the event you're concerned about, let them know your plan, and ask them for support in sticking to your goal. This is the girlfriend who might decide to not drink with you at brunch. Or at the very least, can tell your other friends to lay off if they suck their teeth or roll their eyes at your sobriety. The goal is to make choices in advance around avoidance or allyship so you don't end up in a pressure cooker later.

Real talk: I know there will be moments that you can't predict. Times when you're in a bar and your crowd of friends starts to slowly thin out as everyone steps outside to go smoke. Or when you're in line to get into a restaurant and the host hands you a drink to thank you for patiently waiting to be seated. Now you're in the moment you didn't see coming. You're wondering what you'll do. You could avoid the smoke scene by staying inside the bar or going home. You could ask the host if you can get a free dessert instead of a drink. Or, take this as permission to just say no. It's actually a situation where those three little words from that '80s campaign should and can work.

Mind-Changing Conversation #6: Starting a Cultural Revolution

Now that you've got the three-step plan (recognize, avoid, plan), I want to show you how to use it in some of the most common and complicated situations where substances are baked into our culture.

The Inevitable Teenage Rite of Passage
Maybe this is the first high school party. Or the senior graduation soiree. Whatever the structure, you'll recognize it when it happens. It's the first

announced moment when your kid may have to make choices about what substances they will and won't do while surrounded by their peers.

Get all the information. When my kids are invited to a party, I have a standard list of questions that I ask them: Who will be at the party? Is it chaperoned? Do you think there will be alcohol or other drugs? If yes, how will you manage yourself? All of this sets the foundation for teaching my kids how to recognize potentially difficult environments and decide if they want to avoid them or begin to create a plan to navigate them.

Figure out where you stand. If you're not all right with the idea of a coed sleepover or the weekend party when someone's parents will be away, you're the parent and you've got veto power. But if you do let them go, it's time to set some parameters. In our house, this sounds like:

》 "Your father and I are letting you go to this party because we trust your ability to recognize an unsafe situation and get yourself to safety. I know there's no way of predicting what you could get exposed to there, but I want us to have a plan about how you can avoid things you don't want to be doing. You can keep yourself safe by watching what you eat and drink. If you're drinking out of a punch bowl, you don't really know what's mixed into that bowl. So, stick to bottles and cans you open yourself. If you're eating brownies off the table, you have no idea if it's just dessert or if there's marijuana baked in. Stick to the bags of chips and pretzels. Also, know that I always want you to be honest with me. Your father and I are going to drug screen you when you get home, but you're not going to get into trouble if it comes back positive. If you took something on purpose, just tell us beforehand and we can talk about why you made that choice. If you took something by accident, we want to know that too."

I should note that I can talk to my kids about drug screenings this way because we've normalized drug screenings instead of making them something punitive that only law enforcement does. The narrative in our home has always been that substance use disorders are chronic illnesses; like all illnesses, the earlier we intervene the better; and the first intervention is compassion. They know I view drug screenings no differently from me taking their temperature or oxygen level if they tell me they have a sore throat or trouble catching their breath.

Drug tests are an opportunity for more information that can help our kids protect themselves. If they tell us to expect the drug screen to show nicotine because they were vaping at the party, but marijuana comes up unexpectedly, we have two possible opportunities—create more safety for honesty (like, "Okay, Mom, we were also doing edibles") or ask questions before eating the brownies at Jake's house next party.

Help them create a plan. One of the smartest plans we've come up with is having a safe word or safe phrase our kids can use with us via text to get parachuted out of a situation they don't want to be in. That's avoidance at its best. Because even if you give kids all the right words to say, something about an environment full of friends you want to keep can make you lose your words when you most need them. When we drop our kids off at a party, we let them know that we will stay in the area and they can send us a text if they need to get picked up for any reason. I tell them:

> "I don't care if you're drunk or have taken all the things and are crazy high, text us the code word and we'll get you out of there in fifteen minutes or less. You can just tell your friends there was an emergency at home."

Hilariously, my oldest chose his party safe phrase to be "Mom, I drank the Kool-Aid."

The more tools you can give your kid for avoiding alcohol or drug use under pressure, the better off they'll be. Having a laundry list of options to choose from makes avoiding drugs and alcohol a lot easier.

The Unavoidable and Indulgent Holiday

The holidays are one of the hardest times to set boundaries. We're already using our coping skills to the nth degree to negotiate family dynamics and then substances get introduced into the equation. That might be one of the reasons why New Year's Eve, the Fourth of July, and Thanksgiving are the top three deadliest days of the year for drunk driving. Despite the fact that data shows fatalities spike more than double on New Year's Eve, somehow we haven't been able to reverse the trend.

While you can't be expected to change the behavior of millions of other people across the country (or even the five family members at holiday dinner), you can control how you act and interact with others. Here's a plan:

UN-ADDICTION

Decide how much you want to consume. There's no wrong answer for this. You can decide that you don't want to use any substances at all. You can decide that your cutoff is three drinks or one hit from a bong. The idea is to set your limits beforehand.

Get all the information. The same way that you would ask a kid what to expect at the party, you need to know as well. Try texting your host and asking them if there will be mocktails or spritzers at the event. If not, bring a nonalcoholic beverage (an exotic juice, a flavored sparkling water, unique loose-leaf teas) the same way other guests would automatically bring a bottle of wine. Or if you're going to a restaurant, look up the menu online to see what nonalcoholic beverages you can choose.

Practice your speech. Plan what you'll say when you're offered a substance, so your response comes off effortlessly.

》 "Man, that's tempting but I promised a friend I'd drive him home tonight."

》 "Guess who drew the short straw at work this week? I'm on call for tomorrow and there's no way I want to be responding to emails hungover from tonight."

》 "No thanks. Yours truly has an appointment with her trainer first thing tomorrow. I got serious about getting healthy, so I have to pass."

》 "I got an extension on a paper, but it's due tomorrow. If I get one more bad grade, my parents will kill me, so I'm going to pass. But thanks!"

Give yourself some grace. Boundary-setting bravado doesn't happen overnight. It takes practice, starting with small boundaries (like not taking work calls after hours), and building up to bigger ones (confidently saying "no thank you" to alcohol at the office holiday party). Keep building your boundary-setting muscle and it will get stronger over time.

The Buck Wild Vacation Getaway

As innocuous as it seems, the phrase "When in Rome" has probably gotten just as many people in trouble as "What happens in Vegas, stays in Vegas." A change in environment often gives people permission to take on a different personality. I can just rattle off a list of places and you can imagine how someone might indulge in a way they wouldn't normally: New Orleans and Mardi Gras. Amsterdam. Negril, Jamaica. Coachella Valley. Denver, Colorado. Literally any spring break destination for college kids. Bottom line: Going on vacation can be a significant risk factor for substance use. On one hand, it is totally legitimate to avoid certain destinations that are known for having hard-core partying as part of their culture. But if you want to visit some of those places, here's how you can get on a plane without worrying about getting high (if that's not what you want to do).

Decide how much you want to use. Most people make an unconscious decision to go buck wild on a trip. In that same vein, you can make the conscious decision not to let a trip catapult you into a ten-hour high. Figure out what fun will look like for you and aim for that. You have the right to make that decision to protect your health and your safety.

UN-ADDICTION

Set boundaries. You also have the right not to spend your vacation holding your bestie's hair back as she's kneeling before a toilet after a wild night. That's a kind but firm conversation that you can have with your circle. You might say something like:

> "I know we're all stressed and a lot of us are looking forward to letting loose this vacation, but I'm trying to spend the week by the pool, not in the emergency room. You feel me?"

> "You know I love you all, but the last vacation was a bit much with me staying up all night watching over Danielle. What can we do to make sure that doesn't happen again this trip?"

Pick an ally. Or two. If you're at a holiday party in your hometown and don't want to drink, you may be able to just up and leave. But if you're at a party in another country, that might not feel safe. That's another reason allyship is incredibly important. Pick someone you trust who will be on the trip and share with them the boundaries that you want to set for yourself: Only two drinks a day. Only smoking weed after 6:00 p.m. Definitely no cigarettes. Only trying one new substance. Then let them know how they can intervene if they notice you struggling with those boundaries. If they see you about to order drink number three, how can they compassionately call you out? If they're watching you bum a cigarette off a handsome stranger, what would helping you make a different choice sound like? It could be something along the lines of:

SCROLLING TOWARD ADDICTION

> » "I'm just chiming in here because you told me that you didn't want to get to drink number three. Should we have a mocktail together instead?"

> » "Don't worry, I'm not the Party Police. But we did talk about you not smoking at all this vacation. How can I help you hold to that goal?"

One last point I want to drive home is that if you did decide to, say, stop at drink number two, you haven't missed the goal until drink number three hits your mouth. You have a chance to make a different choice while you're placing the order, while the bartender is mixing it up, and yes, even while you're raising the glass to your mouth. In many recovery programs, people are taught that the moment you consider using a substance, the relapse has already happened. I tell my patients that you haven't used until you have used. It's true that the relapse process starts in your mind, but until it turns into a behavior, you're still substance free. There's always a chance to get off the train—and the more you practice deboarding, the easier it gets.

Un-Addicted: Your Acquired Environmental Risk

Our collective culture and the culture of your family, job, community, or Instagram feed impact your risk of substance use and addiction. You'll never look at national holidays or what we accept as rites of passage again in the same way. Let's take a moment to review what we've covered.

Key Takeaways

> **Your risk of addiction is linked to cultural practices.**
> Once we leave the womb, a significant percentage of our risk of developing addiction is tied to cultural influences such as champagne toasts, kegger parties, celebratory cigars, and tailgating. That risk is also linked to specific family traditions your loved ones may have around drugs and alcohol. Maybe a party at home meant lines of cocaine were on the table or a birthday meant everyone was doing fake and real shots.

> **You're constantly culturally bombarded with temptations.**
> Substance use is baked into American culture wherever you look, from holiday festivities to movies, from magazines to sporting events, and more. It's also impressed upon you on a micro level from family customs that were passed on to you, the work culture you adopt, and the community traditions you engage in.

> **You're capable of creating your own cultural revolution.**
> Just because most Americans toast with champagne to bring in the New Year doesn't mean you have to. Creating new traditions can have a protective benefit for you and your loved ones.

Your Homework

> **Reimagine a ritual.**
> Make a list of the recurring family rituals that you and your loved ones have involving substance use. Then give that event a makeover that doesn't involve drugs or alcohol.

> **Restrict yourself.**
> Try a dry January ... or February ... or ... you get the picture. Experience what it's like to actively avoid alcohol (or not smoke marijuana or not eat edibles) for the next thirty-one days whether you believe you have a problem or not.

> **Rewrite your reactions.**
> The next time someone turns down an alcoholic beverage, don't ask why or request a backstory. Just be supportive. Avoid adding to their frustration or creating shame. Instead, normalize and celebrate their decision not to drink.

> **Take three steps away from the herd.**
> Use the three-step process of recognizing, avoiding, and planning to prevent situations where peer pressure might cause you to make a choice that you wouldn't have otherwise.

Conclusion

Five years ago, I was sitting at my computer cleaning out my LinkedIn inbox, mostly copying and pasting polite "no thank you" responses to a mountain of job recruitment messages. I had been at my job as Chief Medical Officer of a California-based, private, nonprofit behavioral health system for eight years and was curious what other opportunities might be available. Honestly, it didn't seem like there was much to be excited about. The opioid crisis was raging and a constant headline in the media. There was a nationwide sense of urgency to increase access to medications for opioid addiction, but the urgency was focused solely on opioids and not on changing the healthcare system itself in ways that could actually solve the complex root causes of the crisis we were facing.

Message after message in my inbox was from addiction treatment companies trying to recruit me to be their Chief Medical Officer. They touted new medical models to address the opioid crisis. "There isn't enough access," their recruiter or head of human resources would write to me. "Our company will make it easier for people to get the care they so desperately need!" But what they were pitching wasn't new, it was simply an expansion of the current healthcare system that separates physical health from mental health and fails to consider cultural and social needs of people—and delivers record high overdose deaths. How could I feel excited or hopeful about this?

So I No Thank You'd my way to a zero inbox. Until one of the companies I'd just rejected replied back. It was the conversation that changed everything.

CONCLUSION

"Hi Nzinga! Can I ask why you said no thank you to us before hearing more about what we're trying to do?" a woman named Olivia messaged me asking.

So I stepped on my soapbox and sent a long message back.

I explained that a company formed only to address opioid use disorders—and nothing else—would only fail to save lives. I told her that if you want people to get better, you have to care for the whole person because, as you already know, we're not talking about "addicts." We're talking about *people* with addiction. I said there's a difference between treating a diagnosis and caring for a person. I explained that people with opioid use disorders more often than not have other mental and physical health conditions (like anxiety and diabetes) and other needs due to social drivers of health (like access to quality care and support systems). You can't simply isolate and try to cure one concern without addressing all of the others and hope to actually help people get better. I went on to point out that the care model most companies had was short-term and time-limited: five days in detox, three weeks in intensive outpatient, and then good luck. I shared with her what you already know: that addiction is about disconnection. I explained that the environment and lasting support systems that enable and empower people to live life with meaning and purpose were the keys to success—and that's why I would never want to start or run a company that believes creating more access to a fundamentally broken system is the answer.

Olivia didn't skip a beat.

"We're looking for a founding Chief Medical Officer, so that person would be designing the care model. You could address all of those things," she said. "I really think we should talk further."

CONCLUSION

Nine months and two more passionate co-founders later, Eleanor Health was born with the mission to help people affected by addiction live amazing lives. The current standard addiction treatment system focuses on only one of the six pillars I laid out in this book: your acquired biological risk. It prescribes medication for symptoms that have already begun wreaking havoc on your life. At Eleanor, we aim to help our members address all six pillars. We evaluate inherited *and* acquired biological risk factors; we understand the impact of ACEs and the importance of PCEs, including the effect of racism and discrimination; we seek to empower our members to recognize the interplay between the cultures and environments they live in and their health. We do our best to help remove barriers to recovery whether that's finding affordable housing, dealing with financial stress, or overcoming disconnection. Most important, we're committed to helping our community members develop life meaning and purpose as a part of their Magic Formula™ for recovery.

People thought we were being completely unrealistic. What health insurance is going to pay for life meaning and purpose? They told us that, even if we found a health insurance that believed in this approach, we'd never be able to cut through the bureaucratic red tape and redesign a system committed to the way things have always been. I'm happy to say the naysayers were wrong! Now, that is not to say it has all been easy, because it hasn't. Change on an individual level is hard enough—let alone change on a systemic level. But guess what? People's lives are getting better. The people we treat are spending less time in emergency rooms and inpatient hospital units. They report improvements in their physical, mental, social health, and quality of life.

CONCLUSION

Even though we've managed to impact so many lives at Eleanor Health, I know there is still so much to do and there are so many minds to change. There's one statistic that continues to keep me awake at night. Each year, nine out of ten people with a substance use disorder in the United States do not get care. *Nine out of ten.* We have really got to do better. I'm doing my absolute best from *within* the healthcare system. I need your help from *outside* of it. Now that you understand the assignment, are you ready to take it on?

What I've tried to do with this book is to teach you how to have your own powerful conversations to reduce stigma, recognize signs of addiction, and create connections to help yourself and others take action against substance use disorders. In some ways, having these conversations is more important than it ever has been because getting help is still so hard. But imagine if it were easy. Imagine if telling someone you have an addiction was as easy as telling them you had high blood pressure. Imagine if everyone knew about the six pillars that put you at risk for addiction and could talk to you about how your ACEs, experience with discrimination, or your DNA has contributed to risk. Imagine if everyone knew they had a 75 percent chance of recovery instead of shaking their head and telling you it was impossible.

As I finish writing this book, I'm filled with hope and an unwavering belief in the power these pages have to get us on a path to easy. As you read the final words, I hope your perspective about addiction has shifted. I hope that you've seen the power of conversations to make a difference in people's lives and that you go out into the world and use your words for good. And, most of all, I hope that you take this first, critical step (and many more after that) in helping all of us become un-addicted.

Recommended Resources

Apps that help you quit or cut back substance use

Eleanor Health (eleanor.health) Offers wellness, addiction, and mental health education, step-by-step action planning on your health goals, and connection to your Eleanor care team.

I Am Sober (iamsober.com) Track your sobriety with a community that understands what you're going through. Build new daily habits and learn from others who are making changes happen.

QuitNow (quitnow.app/en) Provides a robust community of former smokers to support you on your journey.

SoberTool (sobertool.com) A Harvard-educated licensed alcohol and drug counselor offers in-the-moment craving support for people who want to quit any substance or excessive habit, along with ways for you to measure the progress you're making.

Websites to help you understand addiction

American Academy of Addiction Psychiatry (AAAP) (aaap.org) A professional organization that also offers resources for families and patients including a database of addiction psychiatrists by state, treatment facilities by location, and a resource library where you can find information on everything from dealing with chronic pain to recovery support.

American Society of Addiction Medicine (ASAM) (asam.org) Provides a database of board-certified physicians in addiction medicine, psychiatry, neurology, and more.

Eleanor Health (eleanorhealth.com) Mental health and addiction treatment provider offering compassionate care, a whole-person approach, and evidence-based treatments that are rooted in respect for its community members' values, culture, and life experiences.

National Council for Mental Wellbeing (thenationalcouncil.org) Offers courses in Mental Health First Aid and sponsors programs, events, and courses for professionals across the country.

RECOMMENDED RESOURCES

***Shatterproof** (shatterproof.org)* Provides resources for understanding addiction, finding treatment centers, and paying for treatment. Also provides crisis support for people with addiction as well as friends and family members.

***Substance Abuse and Mental Health Services Administration (SAMHSA)** (samhsa.gov)* This U.S. Department of Health & Human Services site provides multiple sources for treatment facilities and programs in the United States or U.S. territories for mental and substance use disorders. It also includes videos and resources for understanding different substances and addressing mental illness.

Websites for culturally relevant care

***BEAM: Black Emotional and Mental Health Collective** (beam.community)* Provides emotional and mental health resources including hotlines to call, programs to take, wellness tools to use, events to attend, and more.

***Health in Her HUE** (healthinherhue.com)* Health in Her HUE connects Black women and women of color to culturally sensitive healthcare providers, evidence-based health content, and community support.

***Hopscotch Health** (hellohopscotch.com)* On a mission to increase quality of care and access to healthcare for people who live in rural communities.

***Plume** (getplume.co)* For trans people and by trans people, Plume is the largest health provider for the trans and nonbinary community.

Hotlines and Resources

***211** (211.org)* These confidential calls can connect you with resources for mental health, financial support, access to food, and more across the nation.

***988** (988lifeline.org)* A 24-hour suicide and crisis hotline available nationwide.

FindTreatment.gov This U.S. Department of Health & Human Services site offers treatment options for addiction, ideas for how to pay for treatment, and resources for better understanding addiction and mental health.

My Addiction Family Tree

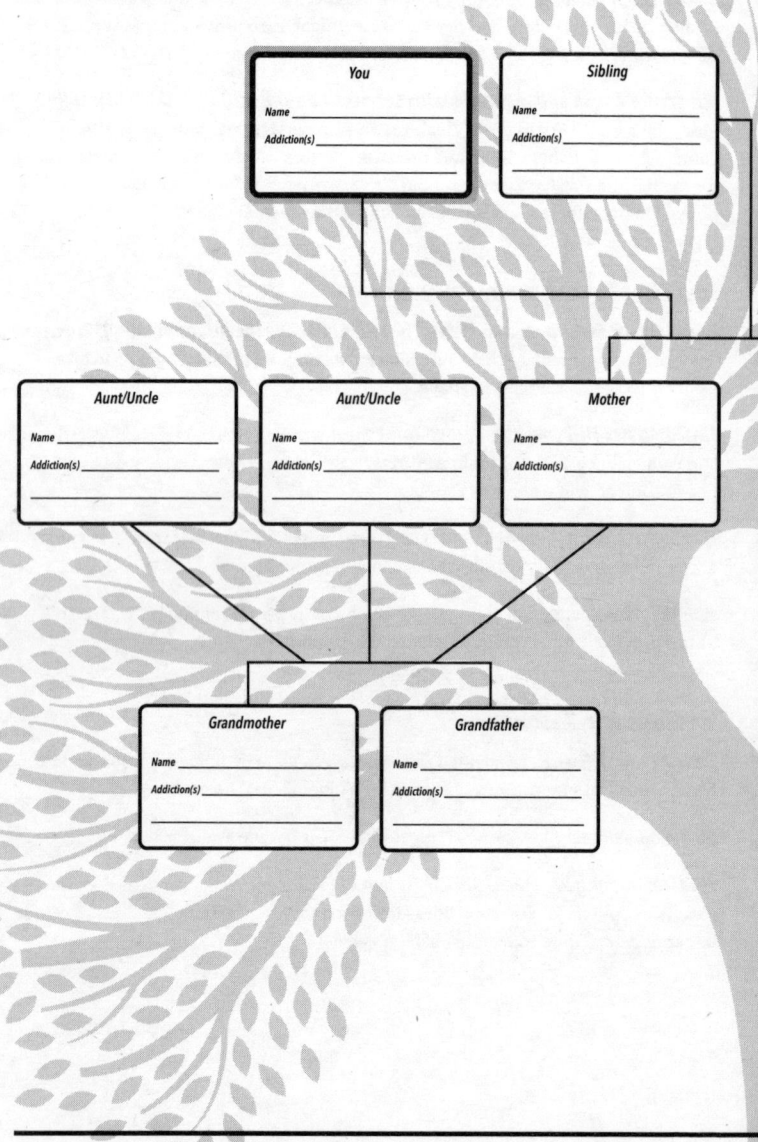

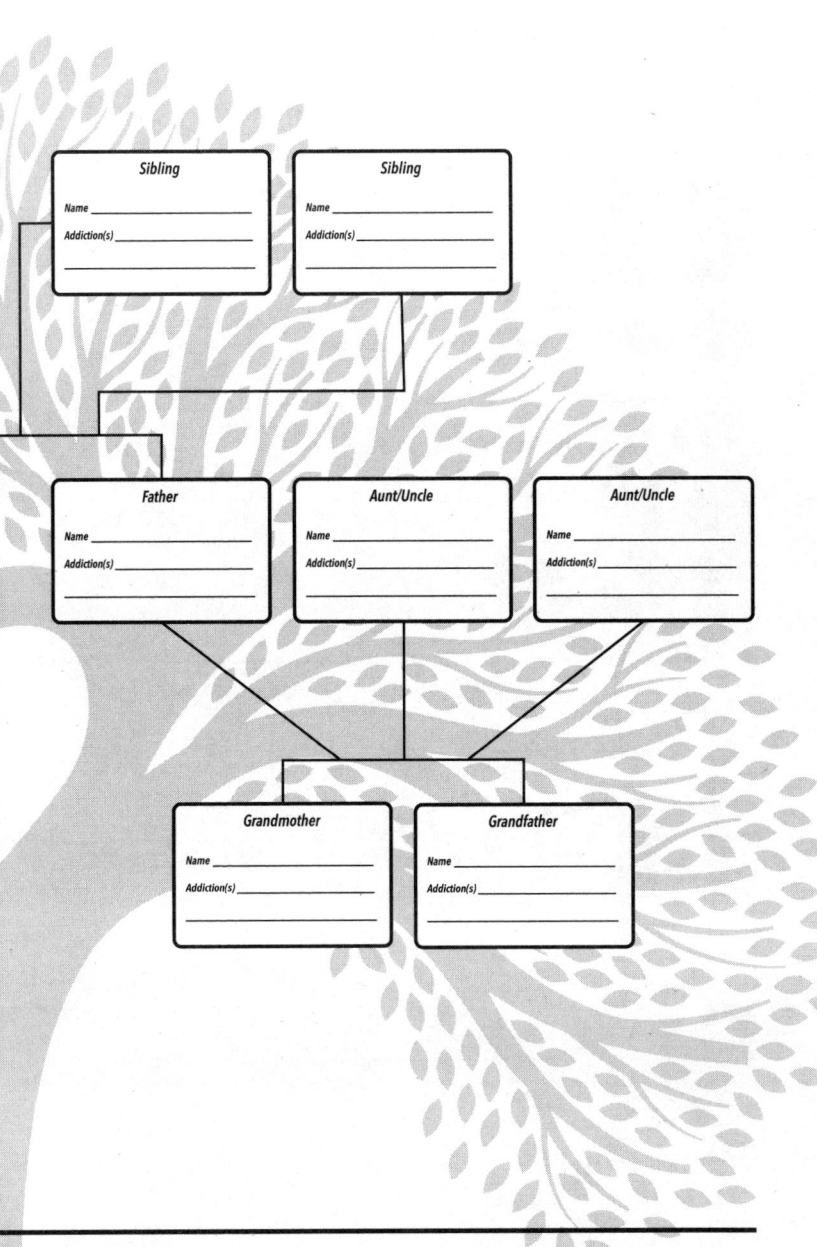

APPENDIX

MM/DD/YYYY

Substance Use Journal

☐ **MONDAY**	**BECAUSE:**	**DESIRE SCALE:**	**MOOD:**
☐ **TUESDAY**	☐ Cravings ☐ Tired	☐ 1 (Low)	🙂
☐ **WEDNESDAY**	☐ Sadness ☐ Social	☐ 2	😐
☐ **THURSDAY**	☐ Unfocused ☐ Anxiety	☐ 3	☹️
	☐ Bored ☐ Curiosity	☐ 4	😓
	☐ _____	☐ 5 (High)	😠

☐ **FRIDAY**

FEELING DIRECTLY BEFORE AND AFTER: _____
_____
_____

☐ **SATURDAY**

FEELING NEXT DAY: _____
_____
_____

☐ **SUNDAY**

TIME: _____ AM / PM

SUBSTANCE(S) USED:
_____
_____
_____

AMOUNT: _____

SLEEP/WAKE TIME: _____

SLEEP QUALITY:
Poor   So-So   Good   Great

EXERCISE: _____

DURATION: _____

DIET:
Poor   So-So   Good   Great

NOTES:
_____
_____

GOALS:
_____
_____

Notes

Preface

x *A full 75 percent of Americans with substance use disorders are in recovery or recovered*: Jones CM, Noonan RK, Compton WM. "Prevalence and correlates of ever having a substance use problem and substance use recovery status among adults in the United States, 2018." *Drug and Alcohol Dependence* 2020;214. https://www.sciencedirect.com/science/article/abs/pii/S0376871620303343

xi *Forty-six percent of adults have a family member or close friend who is or has been addicted to drugs*: "Nearly half of Americans have a family member or close friend who's been addicted to drugs." *Pew Research Center Survey,* 2017. https://www.pewresearch.org/short-reads/2017/10/26/nearly-half-of-americans-have-a-family-member-or-close-friend-whos-been-addicted-to-drugs/

xii *Thirty percent of Americans believe recovery from drug addiction is impossible*: Barry CL, McGinty EE, Pescosolido BA, Goldman HH. "Stigma, discrimination, treatment effectiveness, and policy: public views about drug addiction and mental illness." *Psychiatr Serv* 2014 Oct;65(10):1269–72. https://www.ncbi.nlm.nih.gov/pmc/articles/PMC4285770/

xii *One-year relapse rates for high blood pressure and asthma were the same as or higher than relapse rates for addiction*: McLellan AT, Lewis DC, O'Brien CP, Kleber HD. "Drug Dependence, a Chronic Medical Illness: Implications for Treatment, Insurance, and Outcomes Evaluation." *JAMA* 2000;284(13):1689–95. See page 1693 and Chart in Chapter 1. https://citeseerx.ist.psu.edu/viewdoc/download?doi=10.1.1.462.8284&rep=rep1&type=pdf

Introduction

1 *When I talk about addiction*: "Definition of Addiction." American Society of Addiction Medicine. https://www.asam.org/quality-care/definition-of-addiction

1 *A professional medical society for more than 7,000 physicians, clinicians, and associated professionals . . .* : "About Us." American Society of Addiction Medicine. https://www.asam.org/about-us

2 *When you have an obsessive-compulsive disorder*: "Diseases & Conditions." Mayo Clinic. https://www.mayoclinic.org/diseases-conditions/obsessive-compulsive-disorder/symptoms-causes/syc-20354432

4 *One of the roughly six million children in the United States*: "Asthma in Children." Centers for Disease Control and Prevention. https://www.cdc.gov/vitalsigns/childhood-asthma/index.html

NOTES

5   *Stress then triggers symptoms*: "Emotions, Stress and Depression." Asthma and Allergy Foundation of America. https://aafa.org/asthma/asthma-triggers-causes/emotions-stress-depression/

5   *Which can actually lead to more frequent and worse asthma symptoms*: Gerald JK, Carr TF, Wei CY, Holbrook JT, Gerald LB. "Albuterol Overuse: A Marker of Psychological Distress?" *J Allergy Clin Immunol Pract* 2015 Nov–Dec;3(6):957–62. https://www.ncbi.nlm.nih.gov/pmc/articles/PMC4641773/

6   *Up to 60 percent of the risk of developing a substance use disorder is inherited*: McLellan AT, Lewis DC, O'Brien CP, Kleber HD. "Drug Dependence, a Chronic Medical Illness: Implications for Treatment, Insurance, and Outcomes Evaluation." *JAMA* 2000;284(13):1689–95. https://citeseerx.ist.psu.edu/viewdoc/download?doi=10.1.1.462.8284&rep=rep1&type=pdf

10 *Nearly 70 percent of Americans drank alcohol in the past year. But only 11.3 percent of Americans have an alcohol use disorder*: "Alcohol Facts and Statistics." National Institute on Alcohol Abuse and Alcoholism. https://www.niaaa.nih.gov/publications/brochures-and-fact-sheets/alcohol-facts-and-statistics

11 *Roughly 48 million Americans who smoke marijuana every year ... only 10 percent of those who use marijuana will develop an addiction to it. For regular marijuana users, that number grows to 30 percent, meaning an estimated three of ten regular marijuana users will meet criteria for marijuana use disorder*: "Marijuana and Public Health." Centers for Disease Control and Prevention. https://www.cdc.gov/marijuana/data-statistics.htm | "Addiction (Marijuana or Cannabis Use Disorder)." Centers for Disease Control and Prevention. https://www.cdc.gov/marijuana/health-effects/addiction.html

12 *One survey found that*: Levy AG, Scherer AM, Zikmund-Fisher BJ, Larkin K, Barnes GD, Fagerlin A. "Prevalence of and Factors Associated with Patient Nondisclosure of Medically Relevant Information to Clinicians." *JAMA Netw Open* 2018;1(7):e185293 | "The States That Lie to Their Doctor the Most." Pharmacist.org. www.usarx.com/states-that-lie-to-doctors

14 *Relapse rates are between 7 and 42 percent in the first five years with a higher relapse rate associated with higher stage at time of diagnosis*: "Mayo Clinic Q and A: Reducing your risk of colon cancer." https://newsnetwork.mayoclinic.org/discussion/mayo-clinic-q-and-a-reducing-your-risk-of-colon-cancer-recurrence | Walker AS, Johnson EK, Maykel JA, Stojadinovic A, Nissan A, Brucher B, Champagne BJ, Steele SR. "Future Directions for the Early Detection of Colorectal Cancer Recurrence." *J Cancer* 2014;5(4):272–280. https://www.jcancer.org/v05p0272.htm | Duineveld LA, van Asselt KM, Bemelman WA, Smits AB, Tanis PJ, van Weert HC, Wind J. "Symptomatic and Asymptomatic Colon Cancer Recurrence: A Multicenter Cohort Study." *Ann Fam Med* 2016 May;14(3):215–20. https://www.ncbi.nlm.nih.gov/pmc/articles/PMC4868559/

NOTES

Chapter One: Why Some Monkeys Can't Lay Off the Mojitos

19 *The island's vervet monkey population has developed an interest in alcohol*: "Alcoholic Vervet Monkeys!" BBC Animals, BBC Studios. https://www.youtube.com/watch?v=pSm7BcQHWXk | "Do Animals Like Drugs and Alcohol?" BBC Future. https://www.bbc.com/future/article/20140528-do-animals-take-drugs | "Drunk Monkeys Like Human Party Animals." *New York Post*. https://nypost.com/2002/03/07/drunk-monkeys-like-human-party-animals

21 *We share the majority of our DNA with them*: Pfeifer SP. "The Demographic and Adaptive History of the African Green Monkey." *Molecular Biology and Evolution* 2017;34(5). https://academic.oup.com/mbe/article/34/5/1055/2983514 | "Alcohol can make a monkey out of us." *The Guardian*, April 26, 2011. https://www.theguardian.com/science/punctuated-equilibrium/2011/apr/26/1 | Palmour RM, Mulligan J, Howbert JJ, Ervin F. "Of monkeys and men: vervets and the genetics of human-like behaviors." *Am J Hum Genet* 1997 Sep;61(3):481–8. https://www.ncbi.nlm.nih.gov/pmc/articles/PMC1715973/?page=1

22 *List of chronic illnesses, which the Centers for Disease Control defines...*: "About Chronic Diseases." Centers for Disease Control and Prevention. https://www.cdc.gov/chronicdisease/about/index.htm

23 *Heritability... explains...*: "What is heritability?" MedlinePlus. https://medlineplus.gov/genetics/understanding/inheritance/heritability/

24 *Different addictions are associated with different genes*: Prom-Wormley EC, Ebejer J, Dick DM, Bowers MS. "The genetic epidemiology of substance use disorder: A review." *Drug Alcohol Depend* 2017 Nov 1;180:241–59. https://www.ncbi.nlm.nih.gov/pmc/articles/PMC5911369/; Deak JD, Johnson EC. "Genetics of substance use disorders: a review." *Psychol Med* 2021 Oct;51(13):2189–2200. https://www.ncbi.nlm.nih.gov/pmc/articles/PMC8477224/

31 *Engaging in just five minutes of deep breathing or mindfulness meditation practice can lower your blood pressure*: Manandhar SA, Pramanik T. "Immediate Effect of Slow Deep Breathing Exercise on Blood Pressure and Reaction Time." *Mymensingh Med J* 2019 Oct;28(4):925–9 | Pramanik T, Sharma HO, Mishra S, Mishra A, Prajapati R, Singh S. "Immediate effect of slow pace bhastrika pranayama on blood pressure and heart rate." *J Altern Complement Med* 2009 Mar;15(3):293–5 | "What Does Mindfulness Meditation Do to Your Brain?" *Scientific American*. https://blogs.scientificamerican.com/guest-blog/what-does-mindfulness-meditation-do-to-your-brain/

36 *The DSM-V includes a list of eleven criteria*: Hasin DS, O'Brien CP, Auriacombe M, Borges G, Bucholz K, Budney A, Compton WM, Crowley T, Ling W, Petry NM, Schuckit M, Grant BF. "DSM-5 criteria for substance use disorders: recommendations and rationale." *Am J Psychiatry* 2013 Aug;170(8):834–51. https://www.ncbi.nlm.nih.gov/pmc/articles/PMC3767415/

37 *The term "prediabetes" was coined around 2003 to drive early intervention*: "The war on 'prediabetes' could be a boon for pharma—but is it good medicine?" *Science*. https://www.science.org/content/article/war-prediabetes-could-be-boon-pharma-it-good-medicine

NOTES

37 *There has been a 35 percent decrease in cases of diagnosed diabetes since rates peaked in 2009*: "After 20-Year Increase, New Diabetes Cases Decline." Centers for Disease Control and Prevention. https://www.cdc.gov/diabetes/research/reports/cdc-research-20yr-report.html

37 *It most often takes years to develop*: Marel C, Sunderland M, Mills KL, Slade T, Teesson M, Chapman C. "Conditional probabilities of substance use disorders and associated risk factors: Progression from first use to use disorder on alcohol, cannabis, stimulants, sedatives and opioids." *Drug and Alcohol Dependence* 2019;194:136–42. https://www.sciencedirect.com/science/article/pii/S0376871618305313

37 *Research shows that a brief intervention with your doctor*: Stead LF, Buitrago D, Preciado N, Sanchez G, Hartmann-Boyce J, Lancaster T. "Physician advice for smoking cessation." *Cochrane Database of Systematic Reviews* 2013(5). https://www.cochranelibrary.com/cdsr/doi/10.1002/14651858.CD000165.pub4/full

38 *In addiction medicine, there's another very easy tool for identifying early warning signs for addiction called CAGE*: Malet L, Schwan R, Boussiron D, Aublet-Cuvelier B, Llorca PM. "Validity of the CAGE questionnaire in hospital." *Eur Psychiatry* 2005 Nov;20(7):484–9. https://pubmed.ncbi.nlm.nih.gov/16310679/

43 *The National Institute on Alcohol Abuse and Alcoholism defines heavy drinking*: "Drinking Levels Defined." National Institute on Alcohol Abuse and Alcoholism. https://www.niaaa.nih.gov/alcohol-health/overview-alcohol-consumption/moderate-binge-drinking

Chapter Two: The Accidental Discovery of an Addiction Predictor

57 *Vincent Felitti and ACEs story*: Phone interview with Vincent Felitti, Thursday, October 27, 2022 | "The Adverse Childhood Experiences Study—the largest, most important public health study you never heard of—began in an obesity clinic." ACES Too High News. https://acestoohigh.com/2012/10/03/the-adverse-childhood-experiences-study-the-largest-most-important-public-health-study-you-never-heard-of-began-in-an-obesity-clinic/ | "The Lifelong Effects of Adverse Childhood Experiences (ACEs)." Sealaska Heritage Institute speech. https://www.youtube.com/watch?v=gX7bX4ie-qM

60 *Most of the people surveyed (nearly 70 percent)... and 23.5 percent*: Felitti VJ, Anda RF, Nordenberg D, Edwards V, Koss MP, Marks JS. "Relationship of Childhood Abuse and Household Dysfunction to Many of the Leading Causes of Death in Adults." *The Adverse Childhood Experiences (ACE) Study* 1998 May;14(4):245–58. https://www.ajpmonline.org/article/S0749-3797(98)00017-8/fulltext

60 *A shocking 28.3 percent... and 23.3 percent*: Anda RF, Felitti VJ, Bremner JD, Walker JD, Whitfield C, Perry BD, Dube SR, Giles WH. "The enduring effects of abuse and related adverse experiences in childhood. A convergence of evidence from neurobiology and epidemiology." *Eur Arch Psychiatry Clin Neurosci* 2006 Apr;256(3):174–86. https://www.ncbi.nlm.nih.gov/pmc/articles/PMC3232061/

NOTES

60 *The higher one's ACEs, the more at risk one is for serious health conditions like obesity, diabetes, and heart disease*: Felitti VJ. "The Relation Between Adverse Childhood Experiences and Adult Health: Turning Gold into Lead." *Perm J* 2002 Winter;6(1):44–7. doi: 10.7812/TPP/02.994. PMID:30313011; PMCID:PMC6220625. https://www.ncbi.nlm.nih.gov/pmc/articles/PMC6220625/ | Hillis SD, Anda RF, Felitti VJ, Nordenberg D, Marchbanks PA. "Adverse childhood experiences and sexually transmitted diseases in men and women: a retrospective study." *Pediatrics* 2000 Jul;106(1):E11 | Zhang X, Monnat SM. "Racial/ethnic differences in clusters of adverse childhood experiences and associations with adolescent mental health." *SSM Popul Health* 2021 Dec 16;17:100997.

61 *Through these subsequent studies, they found that certain groups are more likely to have experienced an adverse childhood event*: "We Can Prevent Childhood Adversity." Centers for Disease Control and Prevention. https://vetoviolence.cdc.gov/apps/aces-infographic/home

63 *This concept is neuroplasticity: the brain's ability*: "What Is Neuroplasticity?" VeryWell Mind. https://www.verywellmind.com/what-is-brain-plasticity-2794886

63 *Scientists can look at brain scans of people before and after weeks of meditation*: "When Science Meets Mindfulness." *Harvard Gazette*. https://news.harvard.edu/gazette/story/2018/04/harvard-researchers-study-how-mindfulness-may-change-the-brain-in-depressed-patients/

63 *How mindfulness can change brain activity, increasing the size of the hippocampus (responsible for factual memory) and decreasing the volume of the amygdala (responsible for emotional memory like fear and anxiety)*: Hölzel BK, Carmody J, Vangel M, Congleton C, Yerramsetti SM, Gard T, Lazar SW. "Mindfulness practice leads to increases in regional brain gray matter density." *Psychiatry Res* 2011 Jan 30;191(1):36–43. https://www.ncbi.nlm.nih.gov/pmc/articles/PMC3004979/

64 *That can lead to a suppressed immune system, cardiovascular problems, and even cancer*: Immune system: Dhabhar FS. "Effects of stress on immune function: the good, the bad, and the beautiful." *Immunol Res* 2014 May;58(2–3):193–210. https://pubmed.ncbi.nlm.nih.gov/24798553/ | Cardio problems: Torpy JM, Lynm C, Glass RM. "Chronic Stress and the Heart." *JAMA* 2007;298(14):1722. doi:10.1001/jama.298.14.1722. https://jamanetwork.com/journals/jama/fullarticle/209139 | Cancer: Dai S, Mo Y, Wang Y, Xiang B, Liao Q, Zhou M, Li X, Li Y, Xiong W, Li G, Guo C, Zeng Z. "Chronic Stress Promotes Cancer Development." *Front Oncol* 2020 Aug 19;10:1492. https://www.ncbi.nlm.nih.gov/pmc/articles/PMC7466429/

67 *The ACE Questions*: Felitti VJ, Anda RF, Nordenberg D, Williamson DF, Spitz AM, Edwards V, Koss MP, Marks JS. "Relationship of childhood abuse and household dysfunction to many of the leading causes of death in adults. The Adverse Childhood Experiences (ACE) Study." *Am J Prev Med* 1998 May;14(4):245–58. doi: 10.1016/s0749-3797(98)00017-8. PMID: 9635069 | "About the CDC-Kaiser ACE Study." https://www.cdc.gov/violenceprevention/aces/about.html

NOTES

68 *This non-touching form of child sexual abuse is a newer concept*: "About Child Sexual Abuse." Prevent Child Abuse North Carolina. https://www.preventchildabusenc.org/resource-hub/about-child-sexual-abuse/

75 *The Philadelphia ACE Project*: "About Us." The Philadelphia ACE Project. https://www.philadelphiaaces.org/about-us | "Development of a Childhood Adversity Questionnaire." PowerPoint. https://ldi.upenn.edu/wp-content/uploads/2021/06/Dunn_Development-of-a-Childhood-Adversity-Questionnaire.pdf

78 *According to a 2019 study published in* JAMA Pediatrics: Bethell C, Jones J, Gombojav N, Linkenbach J, Sege R. "Positive Childhood Experiences and Adult Mental and Relational Health in a Statewide Sample: Associations Across Adverse Childhood Experiences Levels." *JAMA Pediatrics*, 2019;173(11). https://jamanetwork.com/journals/jamapediatrics/fullarticle/2749336

78 *The lead author of that study, Christina Bethell, PhD, MPH, was instrumental in getting ACEs questions added to the National Survey of Children's Health*: "2020 National Survey of Children's Health (NSCH)." Data Research Center for Child and Adolescent Health. https://www.childhealthdata.org/docs/default-source/nsch-docs/2020-nsch-guide-to-topics-and-questions_9-14-21.pdf?sfvrsn=63fe5f17_2 | Email exchanges and January 20, 2023, interview with Bethell.

79 *You can still shore up your PCEs as an adult*: University of California—Los Angeles. "Putting Feelings into Words Produces Therapeutic Effects in the Brain." *ScienceDaily*, 22 June 2007. https://www.sciencedaily.com/releases/2007/06/070622090727.htm | Harandi TF, Taghinasab MM, Nayeri TD. "The correlation of social support with mental health: A meta-analysis." *Electron Physician* 2017 Sep 25;9(9):5212–22. https://www.ncbi.nlm.nih.gov/pmc/articles/PMC5633215 | Bethell C, Jones J, Gombojav N, Linkenbach J, Sege R. "Positive Childhood Experiences and Adult Mental and Relational Health in a Statewide Sample: Associations Across Adverse Childhood Experiences Levels." *JAMA Pediatrics* 2019;173(11):e193007. https://www.sciencedirect.com/science/article/pii/S0277953620304408 | "Is having a sense of belonging important?" Mayo Clinic Health System. https://www.mayoclinichealthsystem.org/hometown-health/speaking-of-health/is-having-a-sense-of-belonging-important | Boeder J, Fruiht V, Hwang S, Blanco G, Chan T. "Learning to Love, Work, and Live Your Best Life: Mentoring in Emerging Adulthood Predicts Later Flourishing and Subjective Well-Being." *Emerging Adulthood* 2022;10(5):1222–34. https://journals.sagepub.com/doi/abs/10.1177/21676968211012879?journalCode=eaxa | Pearson AL, Clevenger KA, Horton TH, Gardiner JC, Asana V, Dougherty BV, Pfeiffer KA. "Feelings of safety during daytime walking: associations with mental health, physical activity and cardiometabolic health in high vacancy, low-income neighborhoods in Detroit, Michigan." *Int J Health Geogr* 2021 May 3;20(1):19. https://www.ncbi.nlm.nih.gov/pmc/articles/PMC8091672/

82 *Some studies showing that friendship is even more important than family in determining your happiness and health*: Michigan State University. "Are friends better for us than family?" *ScienceDaily*. www.sciencedaily.com/releases/2017/06/170606090936.htm

82 *Consider which of the five languages speak to your friends*: Chapman G. *The 5 Love Languages: The Secret to Love That Lasts*. Chicago: Northfield Publishing, 2015.

NOTES

84 *Here are the best suggestions I've found*: "How to Make, and Keep, Friends in Adulthood." *New York Times*, October 1, 2022. https://www.nytimes.com/2022/10/01/well/live/how-to-make-friends-adult.html | Expert advice from Dr. Marisa Franco. In Yankovich G. "How to Actually Make Friends as an Adult IRL." *SELF*. https://www.self.com/story/how-to-make-friends-as-adult | Expert advice from Nicholas Epley, PhD. In Burns E. "How to Make Friends as an Adult." *The Cut*. https://www.thecut.com/article/how-to-make-friends-as-an-adult.html | Expert advice from Dr. Kirmayer. In "12 Simple Ways to Make Friends as an Adult." *Reader's Digest*. https://www.rd.com/list/how-to-make-friends-as-an-adult | "Making Friends as an Adult Isn't Easy, but Luckily, We Have 102 Expert-Backed Ways to Do Just That." *Parade*. https://parade.com/1204851/kaitlin-vogel/how-to-make-friends/

Chapter Three: A Garden of Eden for Rats

94 *A Garden of Eden for Rats story*: "Ted and Nora Sterling Prize for Controversy." Bruce K. Alexander. https://www.brucekalexander.com/audio-video/ted-and-nora-sterling-prize-for-controversy | "Rat Park." *VICE Canada*, 2019. https://www.vice.com/en_ca/series/e64vw6/rat-park | Alexander BK, Beyerstein BL, Hadaway PF, Coambs RB. "Effect of Early and Later Colony Housing on Oral Ingestion of Morphine in Rats." *Pharmacology Biochemistry & Behavior* 1981;15:571–6. https://www.brucekalexander.com/pdf/Rat%20Park%201981%20PB&B.pdf | Alexander BK, Coambs RB, Hadaway PF. "The effect of housing and gender on morphine self-administration in rats." *Psychopharmacology (Berl)* 1978 Jul 6;58(2):175–9. https://pubmed.ncbi.nlm.nih.gov/98787 | Hadaway PF, Alexander BK, Coambs RB, et al. "The effect of housing and gender on preference for morphine-sucrose solutions in rats." *Psychopharmacology* 1979;66:87-91. https://link.springer.com/content/pdf/10.1007/BF00431995.pdf | Gage SH, Sumnall HR. "Rat Park: How a rat paradise changed the narrative of addiction." *Addiction* 2019;114:917–22. https://onlinelibrary.wiley.com/action/showCitFormats?doi=10.1111%2Fadd.14481 | "Interview with Jari Chevalier on Living Hero." Bruce K. Alexander. https://www.brucekalexander.com/audio-video/interview-with-jari-chevalier-on-living-hero | "Addiction: The View from Rat Park (2010)." Bruce K. Alexander. https://www.brucekalexander.com/articles-speeches/rat-park/148-addiction-the-view-from-rat-park | "Bruce Alexander—Dislocation Theory of Addiction." YouTube. https://www.youtube.com/watch?v=05FPW4vwinA

94 *Just say no*: "The Story Behind 'This Is Your Brain on Drugs.'" JSTOR Daily. https://daily.jstor.org/the-story-behind-this-is-your-brain-on-drugs/ | "Just Say No." The Ronald Reagan Presidential Foundation and Institute. https://www.reaganfoundation.org/ronald-reagan/nancy-reagan/her-causes/

95 *Skinner box*: "Skinner Box: What Is an Operant Conditioning Chamber?" *Simply Psychology*. https://simplypsychology.org/what-is-a-skinner-box.html

95 *Morphine (which when processed for street sale becomes the opioid drug heroin)*: "Commonly Used Terms." Centers for Disease Control and Prevention (CDC). https://www.cdc.gov/opioids/basics/terms.html | "What's the difference between heroin, fentanyl, morphine and oxycodone?" Drug Policy Alliance. https://drugpolicy.org/drug-facts/difference-heroin-fentanyl-morphine-oxycodone

NOTES

95 *23 percent of people who use heroin develop an addiction*: "Opioid Addiction 2016 Facts & Figures." American Society of Addiction Medicine (ASAM). https://www.asam.org/docs/default-source/advocacy/opioid-addiction-disease-facts-figures.pdf

97 *Almost 100 percent of the time, the rats opened the door*: "Rats Prefer Social Interaction to Heroin or Methamphetamine." National Institute on Drug Abuse (NIH). https://nida.nih.gov/news-events/nida-notes/2019/08/rats-prefer-social-interaction-to-heroin-or-methamphetamine | Venniro M, Zhang M, Caprioli D, et al. "Volitional social interaction prevents drug addiction in rat models." *Nat Neurosci* 2018;21:1520–9. https://www.nature.com/articles/s41593-018-0246-6

97 *In another study published in 2021 in* Frontiers in Behavioral Neuroscience: Smith MA, Cha HS, Griffith AK, Sharp JL. "Social Contact Reinforces Cocaine Self-Administration in Young Adult Male Rats: The Role of Social Reinforcement in Vulnerability to Drug Use." *Frontiers in Behavioral Neuroscience* 2021;15. https://www.frontiersin.org/articles/10.3389/fnbeh.2021.771114

98 *If you lived alone and had a stay-at-home order*: "A Timeline of COVID-19 Developments in 2020." *American Journal of Managed Care* (AJMC). https://www.ajmc.com/view/a-timeline-of-covid19-developments-in-2020

98 *Zoom reported sales were up a whopping 367 percent compared to the same quarter the previous year*: "Zoom Reports Results for Third Quarter Fiscal Year 2021." Zoom Video Communications, Inc. https://investors.zoom.us/news-releases/news-release-details/correction-zoom-reports-results-third-quarter-fiscal-year-2021

98 *One study showed that 81 percent of people in relationships were having as much or more sex than before*: Štulhofer A, Mehulić J, Briken P, Klapilová K, de Graaf H, Carvalheira AA, Löfgren-Mårtenson C, Nobre P, Chollier M, Köse Ö, Elmerstig E, Lançon C, Plášilová L, Schröder J. "Perceived Changes in Sexual Interest and Distress About Discrepant Sexual Interest During the First Phase of COVID-19 Pandemic: A Multi-Country Assessment in Cohabiting Partnered Individuals." *Arch Sex Behav* 2022 Jan;51(1):231–246.

99 *Twenty percent of people reported trying something new in bed*: "The pandemic changed how Americans have sex. Experts explain why." *USA Today*. https://www.usatoday.com/story/life/health-wellness/2021/09/30/sex-how-much-normal-per-week-couples-covid-pandemics-impact/5903902001/

99 *"Something new" included everything from trying a new position to using marijuana or alcohol before sex*: Lehmiller JJ, Garcia JR, Gesselman AN, Mark KP. "Less Sex, but More Sexual Diversity: Changes in Sexual Behavior during the COVID-19 Coronavirus Pandemic." *Leisure Sciences* 2021;43:1–2, 295–304. https://www.tandfonline.com/doi/abs/10.1080/01490400.2020.1774016

NOTES

99 *And those numbers continued to rise in 2021*: "Hot Kink Summer—Lovehoney and Kinsey Institute Researchers Discovered Americans Are Kinkier." Cision PR Newswire. https://www.prnewswire.com/news-releases/hot-kink-summer-lovehoney-and-kinsey-institute-researchers-discovered-americans-are-kinkier-301327893.html

99 *In 2020, 13 percent of Americans said that they started or increased substance use to cope with the stress of the pandemic*: "Substance use during the pandemic." American Psychological Association. https://www.apa.org/monitor/2021/03/substance-use-pandemic

100 *In a first-of-its-kind national study*: "Peers Speak Out: Improving Substance Use Treatment Outcomes During COVID-19." Community Catalyst. https://facesandvoicesofrecovery.org/wp-content/uploads/2021/01/Peers-Speak-Out_FullReport.pdf

104 *85 percent of people age eighteen and older have drunk alcohol at some point in their life*: "Alcohol Use in the United States." National Institute on Alcohol Abuse and Alcoholism (NIH). https://www.niaaa.nih.gov/publications/brochures-and-fact-sheets/alcohol-facts-and-statistics

104 *Half of all people who used an illicit drug in the past year were not diagnosed with a substance use disorder*: "2020 National Survey on Drug Use and Health (NSDUH) Detailed Tables." Substance Abuse and Mental Health Services Administration (SAMHSA). https://www.samhsa.gov/data/sites/default/files/reports/rpt35323/NSDUHDetailedTabs2020v25/NSDUHDetailedTabs2020v25/NSDUHDetTabsSect5pe2020.htm and https://www.samhsa.gov/data/sites/default/files/reports/rpt35323/NSDUHDetailedTabs2020v25/NSDUHDetailedTabs2020v25/NSDUHDetTabsSect1pe2020.htm

105 *The majority of people recover to controlled use, depending on the substance*: "SAMHSA releases 2020 National Survey on Drug Use and Health." Substance Abuse and Mental Health Services Administration (SAMHSA). https://www.samhsa.gov/newsroom/press-announcements/202110260320

107 *Your DNA plays a smaller role of about 30 percent*: Schroeder SA. "We Can Do Better—Improving the Health of the American People." *The New England Journal of Medicine* 2007 Sept 20;357(12):1221–8.

107 *Researchers call this your ZNA*: Glass TA, Bilal U. "Are neighborhoods causal? Complications arising from the 'stickiness' of ZNA." *Soc Sci Med* 2016 Oct;166:244–53. https://pubmed.ncbi.nlm.nih.gov/26830654/ | "The Key to Good Health May Be in Your 'ZNA.'" Haymarket Medical Network. https://www.empr.com/home/features/the-key-to-good-health-may-be-in-your-zna/3/ | "ZNA's the new DNA: How zip codes have drastic impacts on your health." *Salon*. https://www.salon.com/2016/11/12/how-zip-codes-have-an-impact-on-health/

107 *Researchers often look at and refer to zip codes as being the geographic determinant of health as well*: "10 Reasons to use Census Tract Versus ZIP Code Geography & Demographics." ProximityOne. http://proximityone.com/tracts_zips.htm

NOTES

108 *Lowers your chances of getting a high school diploma from 96 percent to 76 percent*: Wodtke GT, Harding DJ, Elwert F. "Neighborhood Effects in Temporal Perspective: The Impact of Long-Term Exposure to Concentrated Disadvantage on High School Graduation." *American Sociological Review* 2011;76(5):713.

109 *The Berlin Wall*: "Berlin Wall." *Britannica*. https://www.britannica.com/topic/Berlin-Wall | "Crossing 96th Street's Great Divide." *New York Times*, June 1, 2013. https://www.nytimes.com/2013/06/02/nyregion/spanning-96th-streets-great-divide.html | "Dividing Line Between Upper East Side and Harlem Blurring." DNA Info. https://www.dnainfo.com/new-york/20110804/upper-east-side/dividing-line-between-upper-east-side-harlem-blurring/

110 *It marked how long you could expect to live*: "Large Life Expectancy Gaps in U.S. Cities Linked to Racial & Ethnic Segregation by Neighborhood." NYU Langone Health. https://nyulangone.org/news/large-life-expectancy-gaps-us-cities-linked-racial-ethnic-segregation-neighborhood

110 *More than a hundred years*: "Census Tracts." United States Census Bureau. https://www2.census.gov/geo/pdfs/education/CensusTracts.pdf

110 *City Health Project and United States Small-Area Life Expectancy Project*: "United States Small-Area Life Expectancy Estimates Project: Methodology and Results Summary." National Center for Health Statistics (NCHS). https://www.cdc.gov/nchs/pressroom/press_release_usaleep.pdf

110 *A few blocks in one direction could take up to thirty years off your life.*: "Your Zip Code Could Affect Your Lifespan. These Maps Show How." NYU Langone Health. https://www.cityhealthdashboard.com/blog-media/1107

110 *Life expectancy of 66.2 years*: "Metric Detail for Life Expectancy in 2015." NYU Langone Health. https://www.cityhealthdashboard.com/ny/new%20york/metric-detail?metric=837&dataRange=city&metricYearRange=2015%2C+6+Year+Modeled+Estimate

110 *Residents can expect to live 80.9 years*: "Atlanta Population's Life Expectancy Varies by Zip Code." WABE Atlanta. https://www.wabe.org/atlanta-populations-life-expectancy-varies-zip-code/

111 *The neighborhoods of Streeterville and Englewood*: "Your Zip Code Could Affect Your Lifespan. These Maps Show How." NYU Langone Health. https://www.cityhealthdashboard.com/blog-media/1107 | "Chicago's lifespan gap: Streeterville residents live to 90. Englewood residents die at 60. Study finds it's the largest divide in the U.S." *Chicago Tribune*. https://www.chicagotribune.com/business/ct-biz-chicago-has-largest-life-expectancy-gap-between-neighborhoods-20190605-story.html

111 *Twelve-step programs*: "12 Step Programs: 12 Steps to Recovery for Addiction." American Addiction Centers. https://americanaddictioncenters.org/rehab-guide/12-step

NOTES

112 *Increases a teenager's likelihood of drinking alcohol*: Berke EM, Tanski SE, Demidenko E, Alford-Teaster J, Shi X, Sargent JD. "Alcohol retail density and demographic predictors of health disparities: a geographic analysis." *Am J Public Health* 2010 Oct;100(10):1967–71. https://www.ncbi.nlm.nih.gov/pmc/articles/PMC2936987/

112 *Research has shown higher rates of pedestrian injuries and drunk driving accidents*: Watts RK, Rabow J. "Alcohol availability and alcohol-related problems in 213 California cities." *Alcohol Clin Exp Res* 1983 Winter;7(1):47–58. https://pubmed.ncbi.nlm.nih.gov/6342449/ | Scribner RA, MacKinnon DP, Dwyer JH. "Alcohol outlet density and motor vehicle crashes in Los Angeles County cities." *J Stud Alcohol* 1994 Jul;55(4):447–53. https://pubmed.ncbi.nlm.nih.gov/7934052/

112 *One study looked at more than 1,600 zip codes in California to determine that*: Freisthler B, Gruenewald P, Ring L, LaScala E. "An Ecological Assessment of the Population and Environmental Correlates of Childhood Accident, Assault, and Child Abuse Injuries. Alcoholism: Clinical and experimental research." 2008;32(11):1969–75. https://www.ncbi.nlm.nih.gov/pmc/articles/PMC2588484/

113 *High levels of places to buy tobacco in a neighborhood resulted*: Henriksen L, Feighery E, Schleicher N, Cowling D, Kline R, Fortmann S. "Is adolescent smoking related to the density and proximity of tobacco outlets and retail cigarette advertising near schools?" *Preventive Medicine* 2008;47(210):4. https://www.researchgate.net/publication/5311739

113 *An increase in the number of medical cannabis dispensaries in an area*: Mair C, Sumetsky N, Kranich C, Freisthler B. "Availability of medical cannabis dispensaries and cannabis abuse/dependence-related hospitalizations in California." *Addiction* 2021 Jul;116(7):1908–13. https://pubmed.ncbi.nlm.nih.gov/33565655/

114 *The study found that the teens' amygdalae*: "Living with Neighborhood Violence May Shape Teens' Brains." *Scientific American*, June 15, 2018. https://www.scientificamerican.com/article/living-with-neighborhood-violence-may-shape-teens-rsquo-brains/

114 *Research on the children of Holocaust survivors*: Kellermann NP. "Epigenetic transmission of Holocaust trauma: can nightmares be inherited?" *Isr J Psychiatry Relat Sci* 2013;50(1):33–9. https://pubmed.ncbi.nlm.nih.gov/24029109 | "Study finds epigenetic changes in children of Holocaust survivors." U.S. Department of Veterans Affairs. https://www.research.va.gov/currents/1016-3.cfm

114 *1994 Moving to Opportunity study*: "Why Living in a Poor Neighborhood Can Change Your Biology." *Nautilus*. https://nautil.us/why-living-in-a-poor-neighborhood-can-change-your-biology-rp-235731/ | Ludwig J, Sanbonmatsu L, Gennetian L, Adam E, Duncan GJ, Katz LF, Kessler RC, Kling JR, Lindau ST, Whitaker RC, McDade TW. "Neighborhoods, obesity, and diabetes—a randomized social experiment." *New England Journal of Medicine* 2011 Oct 20;365(16):1509–19. https://www.ncbi.nlm.nih.gov/pmc/articles/PMC3410541/

NOTES

120 *Taking a long walk in the park after dinner every night to reduce stress*: "1-hour walk through nature lowers stress, research shows." *Medical News Today*. https://www.medicalnewstoday.com/articles/1-hour-walk-through-nature-lowers-stress-research-shows

Chapter Four: Is Finding a Man the Solution for Jan?

129 *In 1970, if you were a doctor opening up the April issue of the* Archives of General Psychiatry: See opening pages of ads immediately following the table of contents. "35 and Single." *Archives of General Psychiatry* 1970 Apr;22(4), opening pages of ads.

131 *Valium became known as the "white-collar aspirin," "Mother's Little Helper," as the Rolling Stones called it in a song, and "Executive Excedrin."*: Herzberg D. "'The Pill You Love Can Turn on You': Feminism, Tranquilizers, and the Valium Panic of the 1970s." *American Quarterly* 2006;58(1):79–103. http://www.jstor.org/stable/40068349 | "Mother's Little Helper Turns 40." *CBS News*. https://www.cbsnews.com/news/mothers-little-helper-turns-40/ | Associated Press. "Senate Panel Is Told of Dangers of Valium Abuse." *New York Times*, September 11, 1979, Section A, Page 18. https://www.nytimes.com/1979/09/11/archives/senate-panel-is-told-of-dangers-of-valium-abuse-a-nightmare-of.html

132 *Acquired biological risk can come straight from your primary care physician*: "Healthtalk: The '70s Feel-Good Pills and the '80s Addicts." *Washington Post*. https://www.washingtonpost.com/archive/lifestyle/1979/11/30/healthtalk-the-70s-feel-good-pills-and-the-80s-addicts/fff30d24-0b73-4ecd-98ad-21b429633a47/

133 *Up to 40 percent of American adults report insomnia symptoms in a given year*: "Insomnia Overview: Epidemiology, Pathophysiology, Diagnosis and Monitoring, and Nonpharmacologic Therapy." *American Journal of Managed Care* (AJMC). https://www.ajmc.com/view/insomnia-overview-epidemiology-pathophysiology-diagnosis-and-monitoring-and-nonpharmacologic-therapy

133 *About one in three Americans (31.1 percent exactly) have or will experience an anxiety disorder at one point in their lives*: "Any Anxiety Disorder." National Institute of Mental Health (NIH). https://www.nimh.nih.gov/health/statistics/any-anxiety-disorder

133 *When we think about anxiety, we think about the ways it shows up in someone's life both physically and psychologically*: "Anxiety Disorders." National Institute of Mental Health (NIH). https://www.nimh.nih.gov/health/topics/anxiety-disorders | "Anxiety Disorders." Mayo Clinic. https://www.mayoclinic.org/diseases-conditions/anxiety/symptoms-causes/syc-20350961 | "Anxiety Disorders." Cleveland Clinic. https://my.clevelandclinic.org/health/diseases/9536-anxiety-disorders

134 *Sometimes referred to as "daytime tranquilizers."*: "Mother's Little Helper at 50." Massachusetts General Hospital *Proto* magazine. https://protomag.com/medical-history/anniversary-valium-turns-50/

NOTES

135 *The first benzodiazepine, Librium, was accidentally discovered in 1955*: Wick JY. "The history of benzodiazepines." *Consult Pharm* 2013 Sep;28(9):538–48. https://pubmed.ncbi.nlm.nih.gov/24007886/

135 *quickly followed by Valium, which was released a year after a famous blond bombshell's death*: "From the Archives: Marilyn Monroe Dies; Pills Blamed." *Los Angeles Times*. https://www.latimes.com/local/obituaries/archives/la-me-marilyn-monroe-19620806-story.html | "Marilyn Monroe and the prescription drugs that killed her." *PBS Thirteen*. https://www.pbs.org/newshour/health/marilyn-monroe-and-the-prescription-drugs-that-killed-her | "Mother's Little Helper: The History of Valium." History Hit. https://www.historyhit.com/mothers-little-helper-the-history-of-valium/

135 *Plus, benzodiazepines were also an effective treatment for anxiety that hadn't responded to other medications in the past*: "Are Benzodiazepines the New Opioids?" Yale Medicine. https://www.yalemedicine.org/news/benzodiazepine-epidemic

135 *Valium became the first $100 million brand the pharmaceutical industry had ever seen. So many millions of prescriptions were doled out that it became the best-selling medication in the United States between 1968 and 1982*: "Mother's Little Helper at 50." Massachusetts General Hospital *Proto* magazine. https://protomag.com/medical-history/anniversary-valium-turns-50/ | "Americans are spending almost half a billion dollars a year on a drug to relieve their anxiety—a fact that is in itself considerable cause for anxiety." *New York Times*, February 1, 1976. https://www.nytimes.com/1976/02/01/archives/article-16-no-title-americans-are-spending-almost-half-a-billion.html | "Just Saying No to Valium," *JSTOR Daily*, https://daily.jstor.org/just-saying-no-to-valium/

136 *Some experts think that the luster of Valium wore off when*: "Mother's Little Helper at 50." Massachusetts General Hospital *Proto* magazine. https://protomag.com/medical-history/anniversary-valium-turns-50/

138 *By 2013, prescriptions for benzodiazepines were being handed out at the rate of 135 million per year. Over a seventeen-year period, the number of prescriptions had increased by 67 percent and the amount of those prescriptions was up by 300 percent. Unfortunately, the number of overdose deaths from the drug spiked as well, by a stunning 400+ percent*: "Are Benzodiazepines the New Opioids?" *Yale Medicine*, December 11, 2019. https://www.yalemedicine.org/news/benzodiazepine-epidemic | Bachhuber MA, Hennessy S, Cunningham CO, Starrels JL. "Increasing Benzodiazepine Prescriptions and Overdose Mortality in the United States, 1996–2013." *Am J Public Health* 2016 Apr;106(4):686–8. https://pubmed.ncbi.nlm.nih.gov/26890165/ | "There's a New Drug Crisis Harming Americans." *The Hill*, September 25, 2018. https://thehill.com/opinion/healthcare/408350-theres-a-new-drug-crisis-harming-americans/

138 *In 2007, you had Lil Wayne singing about mingling with the stars, throwing a party on Mars, and being a prisoner locked up behind Xanax bars. In 2012, our Brown bombshell, Whitney

NOTES

Houston, accidentally drowned in a bathtub with a mix of drugs, including Xanax, in her system: "I Feel Like Dying" lyrics and release date: June 1, 2007. Genius.com. https://genius.com/Lil-wayne-i-feel-like-dying-lyrics | "Whitney Houston Drowned, Coroner Says." *New York Times*, March 22, 2012. https://www.nytimes.com/2012/03/23/arts/music/whitney-houston-drowned-coroner-says.html

139 *In 2016, the number of prescriptions was declining*: "FDA Holds Workshop to Discuss the Safe Use of Benzodiazepines." U.S. Food & Drug Administration (FDA). https://www.fda.gov/drugs/news-events-human-drugs/fda-holds-workshop-discuss-safe-use-benzodiazepines

139 *The number of teenagers with substance use disorders related to benzodiazepines was on the rise*: "Teen Xanax Abuse Is Surging." The Pew Charitable Trusts. https://www.pewtrusts.org/en/research-and-analysis/blogs/stateline/2018/08/24/teen-xanax-abuse-is-surging

139 *By March of 2020, anxiety and prescriptions for it were back on the rise and everyone from the FDA to scientists are sounding the alarm bell to try to avoid disaster*: Milani SA, Raji MA, Chen L, Kuo Y. "Trends in the Use of Benzodiazepines, Z-Hypnotics, and Serotonergic Drugs Among US Women and Men Before and During the COVID-19 Pandemic." *JAMA Netw Open* 2021;4(10):e2131012. https://jamanetwork.com/journals/jamanetworkopen/fullarticle/2785392 | de Dios C, Fernandes BS, Whalen K, Bandewar S, Suchting R, Weaver MF, Selvaraj S. "Prescription fill patterns for benzodiazepine and opioid drugs during the COVID-19 pandemic in the United States." *Drug Alcohol Depend* 2021 Dec 1;229(Pt A):109176. https://www.ncbi.nlm.nih.gov/pmc/articles/PMC8595244/

140 *Roughly three out of four people who became addicted to illicit opioids (like heroin) started out taking prescription opioids*: "Opioids." Johns Hopkins Medicine. https://www.hopkinsmedicine.org/health/treatment-tests-and-therapies/opioids

140 *Ninety-one people die every day from an opioid overdose*: "Ongoing emergencies & disasters." Centers for Medicare & Medicaid Services (CMS). https://www.cms.gov/about-cms/agency-information/emergency/epro/current-emergencies/ongoing-emergencies

140 *You might be sent home from the hospital with some Vicodin*: Peahl AF, Dalton VK, Montgomery JR, Lai Y, Hu HM, Waljee JF. "Rates of New Persistent Opioid Use After Vaginal or Cesarean Birth Among US Women." *JAMA Netw Open* 2019;2(7):e197863. https://jamanetwork.com/journals/jamanetworkopen/fullarticle/2739048

141 *put him at serious risk for overdosing*: "FDA warns about serious risks and death when combining opioid pain or cough medicines with benzodiazepines; requires its strongest warning." U.S. Food & Drug Administration (FDA). https://www.fda.gov/media/99761/download

141 *One in three American adults with arthritis filled an opioid prescription at a pharmacy in 2015*: "Arthritis and Joint Pain Management." Centers for Disease Control and Prevention (CDC). https://www.cdc.gov/arthritis/pain/joint-pain-management.htm

NOTES

142 *Less than 2 percent of Americans have a prescription opioid use disorder*: "What is the scope of prescription drug misuse in the United States?" National Institute on Drug Abuse (NIDA). https://nida.nih.gov/publications/research-reports/misuse-prescription-drugs/what-scope-prescription-drug-misuse

142 *ADHD meds when used as prescribed to treat ADHD don't increase your risk of substance use disorder*: "Research Shows ADHD Meds Do Not Increase Substance Use Risks." Children and Adults with Attention-Deficit/Hyperactivity Disorder (CHADD). https://chadd.org/adhd-weekly/research-shows-adhd-meds-do-not-increase-substance-use-risks/

143 *Because even though the stimulant overuse epidemic is less recognized, it's still on the rise*: "Experts Warn of Emerging 'Stimulant Epidemic.'" WebMD. https://www.webmd.com/mental-health/addiction/news/20180403/experts-warn-of-emerging-stimulant-epidemic

143 *While less than 2 percent of the population has used cocaine in the past year*: "What is the scope of cocaine use in the United States?" National Institute on Drug Abuse (NIDA). https://nida.nih.gov/publications/research-reports/cocaine/what-scope-cocaine-use-in-united-states | "Stimulants." University of California, Davis. https://shcs.ucdavis.edu/health-topic/stimulants

144 *Benzodiazepine description*: "Benzodiazepines (Benzos)." Cleveland Clinic. https://my.clevelandclinic.org/health/treatments/24570-benzodiazepines-benzos | "Benzodiazepines Drug Fact Sheet." United States Drug Enforcement Administration (DEA). https://www.dea.gov/sites/default/files/2020-06/Benzodiazepenes-2020_1.pdf

144 *Opioid description*: "Get Informed." Centers for Disease Control and Prevention (CDC). https://www.cdc.gov/rxawareness/information/index.html | "Opioids." Johns Hopkins Medicine. https://www.hopkinsmedicine.org/health/treatment-tests-and-therapies/opioids

144 *Stimulants description*: "Stimulants." United States Drug Enforcement Administration (DEA). https://www.dea.gov/taxonomy/term/346 | "Prescription Stimulants DrugFacts." National Institute on Drug Abuse (NIDA). https://nida.nih.gov/publications/drugfacts/prescription-stimulants

146 *A runner's high releases feel-good chemicals, just like opioids work the endorphin receptors in your brain*: "The Truth Behind 'Runner's High' and Other Mental Benefits of Running." Johns Hopkins Medicine. https://www.hopkinsmedicine.org/health/wellness-and-prevention/the-truth-behind-runners-high-and-other-mental-benefits-of-running | "How Opioid Addiction Occurs." Mayo Clinic. https://www.mayoclinic.org/diseases-conditions/prescription-drug-abuse/in-depth/how-opioid-addiction-occurs/art-20360372

149 *Original Opioid Risk Tool*: Webster LR, Webster RM. "Predicting Aberrant Behaviors in Opioid-Treated Patients: Preliminary Validation of the Opioid Risk Tool." *Pain Med* 2005 Nov;6(6):432–42. https://doi.org/10.1111/j.1526-4637.2005.00072.x | "Opioid Risk Tool." https://nida.nih.gov/sites/default/files/opioidrisktool.pdf

NOTES

149 *Icahn School of Medicine description*: "About the School." Icahn School of Medicine at Mount Sinai. https://icahn.mssm.edu/about

149 *In search of answers to a pressing question about cocaine use*: Parvaz MA, Moeller SJ, d'Oleire Uquillas F, Pflumm A, Maloney T, Alia-Klein N, Goldstein RZ. "Prefrontal gray matter volume recovery in treatment-seeking cocaine-addicted individuals: a longitudinal study." *Addict Biol* 2017 Sep;22(5):1391–1401. https://www.ncbi.nlm.nih.gov/pmc/articles/PMC5085900/

150 *The Iowa Gambling Task*: "The Iowa Gambling Task—What Does It Tell Us About the Brain?" iMotions A/S. https://imotions.com/blog/insights/research-insights/iowa-gambling-task/ | "Iowa Gambling Task." PsyToolkit. https://www.psytoolkit.org/experiment-library/igt.html

151 *25 percent of people who are lost to substance use disorders . . . 20 million Americans in recovery*: Jones CM, Noonan RK, Compton WM. "Prevalence and correlates of ever having a substance use problem and substance use recovery status among adults in the United States, 2018." *Drug and Alcohol Dependence* 2020;214. https://www.sciencedirect.com/science/article/abs/pii/S0376871620303343 | "SAMHSA Announces National Survey on Drug Use and Health (NSDUH) Results Detailing Mental Illness and Substance Use Levels in 2021." Health and Human Services. https://www.hhs.gov/about/news/2023/01/04/samhsa-announces-national-survey-drug-use-health-results-detailing-mental-illness-substance-use-levels-2021.html

153 *Due to federal laws currently in place, it is illegal*: "To break down barriers to addiction care, modernize the rules for sharing those medical records." *The Hill*. https://thehill.com/opinion/congress-blog/3621603-to-break-down-barriers-to-addiction-care-modernize-the-rules-for-sharing-those-medical-records/

155 *People with chronic lower back pain are more likely*: Shmagel A, MD; Krebs E, MD, MPH; Ensrud K, MD, MPH; Foley R, MD, FRCPI, FRCPC. "Illicit Substance Use in US Adults With Chronic Low Back Pain." *SPINE* 41(17):1372–77. https://journals.lww.com/spinejournal/Fulltext/2016/09010/Illicit_Substance_Use_in_US_Adults_With_Chronic.13.aspx | Wolters Kluwer Health. "Chronic low back pain linked to higher rates of illicit drug use." *ScienceDaily*. www.sciencedaily.com/releases/2016/07/160721143900.htm

155 *Another study looked at over a thousand veterans*: Vasudevan VN, MD; Black RD, BS; Bowman B, MD; Solomon SS, MD. "Does Subclinical Hyperthyroidism Predispose to Cocaine Addiction?" *Endocr Pract* 2012 Jul;18(4):478–82. https://www.endocrinepractice.org/article/S1530-891X(20)43042-3/fulltext

Chapter Five: How Weathering Any Storm Can Wither Your Health

165 *Geronimus background story*: Phone Interview with Geronimus, January 20, 2023 | "Arline Geronimus: Q&A About Weathering, or How Chronic Stress Prematurely Ages Your Body." *Everyday Health*. https://www.everydayhealth.com/wellness/united-states-of-stress/advisory-board/arline-t-geronimus-q-a/ | "Making The Case That Discrimination Is Bad For Your

NOTES

Health." Code Sw!tch. https://www.npr.org/sections/codeswitch/2018/01/14/577664626/making-the-case-that-discrimination-is-bad-for-your-health | Villarosa L. *Under the Skin: The Hidden Toll of Racism on American Lives and on the Health of Our Nation*. New York: Doubleday, 2022.

166 *Newspaper headlines about Geronimus*: "Study Finds Poor Teens Better Off With Babies." *Salina Journal*, Kansas, February 17, 1990 | "Teen Pregnancy OK for Poor, Says Study." *Chicago Sun-Times*, February 18, 1990 | "Buying Into White Supremacy." *Washington Post*, May 31, 1991.

168 *allostatic load, a term coined by neuroscientist Bruce McEwen and psychologist Eliot Stellar*: "Bruce McEwen, 81, Is Dead; Found Stress Can Alter the Brain." *New York Times*, February 10, 2020. https://www.nytimes.com/2020/02/10/science/bruce-s-mcewen-dead.html | Hill MN, Karatsoreos IN, de Kloet ER, et al. "In memory of Bruce McEwen: a gentle giant of neuroscience." *Nat Neurosci* 2020(23):473–4. https://www.nature.com/articles/s41593-020-0613-y | "Bruce McEwen, Stress Hormone Researcher, Dies." *The Scientist*. https://www.the-scientist.com/news-opinion/bruce-mcewen-stress-hormone-researcher-dies-66918 | McEwen BS, Stellar E. "Stress and the individual. Mechanisms leading to disease." *Arch Intern Med* 1993 Sep 27;153(18):2093–101. https://pubmed.ncbi.nlm.nih.gov/8379800/#affiliation-1 | "Dr. Eliot Stellar, 73; Viewed Psychology Through Physiology." *New York Times*, October 15, 1993. https://www.nytimes.com/1993/10/15/obituaries/dr-eliot-stellar-73-viewed-psychology-through-physiology.html

168 *using allostatic loads, Geronimus found*: Geronimus AT, Hicken M, Keene D, Bound J. "'Weathering' and age patterns of allostatic load scores among blacks and whites in the United States." *American Journal of Public Health* 2006 May;96(5):826–33. https://www.ncbi.nlm.nih.gov/pmc/articles/PMC1470581/

168 *Years later in 2009, molecular biologist Elizabeth Blackburn*: Rogers, K. "Elizabeth Blackburn." *Encyclopedia Britannica*. https://www.britannica.com/biography/Elizabeth-Blackburn | "Elizabeth Blackburn Nobel Prize in Physiology or Medicine 2009." The Nobel Prize. https://www.nobelprize.org/womenwhochangedscience/stories/elizabeth-blackburn

169 *One study of more than 330 Black teens in the rural South*: "Racial Discrimination in Teen Years Could Create Health Problems." *NBC News*. https://www.nbcnews.com/health/health-news/racial-discrimination-teen-years-could-create-health-problems-n20276

170 *felt more like you were trying to punch your way through a concrete roof*: "The Concrete Ceiling." Stanford Social Innovation Review (SSIR). https://ssir.org/articles/entry/the_concrete_ceiling | "REAL Conversations: Breaking Through the Glass and Concrete Ceilings." University of Rochester. https://www.rochester.edu/advancement/wp-content/uploads/2021/03/Resources1.pdf

170 *what some experts call a "glass cliff"*: Ryan MK, Haslam SA. "The Glass Cliff: Evidence that Women are Over-Represented in Precarious Leadership Positions." *British Journal of*

NOTES

Management 2005;16:81–90. https://onlinelibrary.wiley.com/doi/abs/10.1111/j.1467-8551.2005.00433.x | "Studies Show Women & Minority Leaders Have Shorter Tenures, Tenuous Support." *Utah State Today.* https://www.usu.edu/today/story/studies-show-women-amp-minority-leaders-have-shorter-tenures-tenuous-support | "The 'glass cliff': How women and people of color are set up to fail in the workplace." *USA Today.* https://www.today.com/tmrw/glass-cliff-why-women-people-color-are-often-set-fail-t189060 | "The 'glass cliff' is a serious problem for women in corporate America. Here's how to dismantle it." Insider Inc. https://www.businessinsider.com/women-and-people-of-color-face-glass-cliff-us-2020-7

174 *While research has found that racism can lead to increased substance use*: Neblett EW Jr, Terzian M, Harriott V. "From racial discrimination to substance use: the buffering effects of racial socialization." *Child Dev Perspect* 2010;4(2):131–7. https://www.ncbi.nlm.nih.gov/pmc/articles/PMC3674554/ | Gibbons FX, O'Hara RE, Stock ML, Gerrard M, Weng C-Y, Wills TA. "The erosive effects of racism: reduced self-control mediates the relation between perceived racial discrimination and substance use in African American adolescents." *J Pers Soc Psychol* 2012;102(5):1089–1104. https://pubmed.ncbi.nlm.nih.gov/22390225/ | Berger M, Sarnyai Z. "'More than skin deep': stress neurobiology and mental health consequences of racial discrimination." *Stress* 2015;18(1):1–10. https://pubmed.ncbi.nlm.nih.gov/25407297/

175 *In the past year, 70.3 percent of Whites drank compared to*: "Racial/Ethnic Differences in Substance Use, Substance Use Disorders, and Substance Use Treatment Utilization among People Aged 12 or Older (2015–2019)." Substance Abuse and Mental Health Services Administration (SAMHSA). https://www.samhsa.gov/data/sites/default/files/reports/rpt35326/2021NSDUHSUChartbook102221B.pdf

175 *while Black women are 4 percent less likely to develop breast cancer*: "Breast Cancer Death Rates Are Highest for Black Women—Again." American Cancer Society. https://www.cancer.org/latest-news/breast-cancer-death-rates-are-highest-for-black-women-again.html

175 *while Blacks have a far lower incidence rate of skin cancer than Whites*: "Melanoma Among Non-Hispanic Black Americans." Centers for Disease Control and Prevention (CDC). https://www.cdc.gov/pcd/issues/2019/18_0640.htm

175 *Black people have lower rates of substance use disorders overall, but once we have a substance use disorder, we're more likely to lose our job as a result of it or go to prison because of it, more likely to acquire another disease like cirrhosis of the liver because of it, and even more likely to die from it*: "Racial/Ethnic Differences in Substance Use, Substance Use Disorders, and Substance Use Treatment Utilization among People Aged 12 or Older (2015–2019)." Department of Health and Human Services, Substance Abuse and Mental Health Services Administration, Figure 4.7. https://www.samhsa.gov/data/sites/default/files/reports/rpt35326/2021NSDUHSUChartbook102221B.pdf | Farahmand P, MD, MA; Arshed A, MD, MS, MHA; Bradley MV, MD, MS. "Systemic Racism and Substance Use Disorders." *J Psychiatric Annals* 2020;50(11):494–8. https://journals.healio.com/doi/abs/10.3928/00485713-20201008-01

NOTES

176 *Physicians, for example, who go into profession-related recovery programs have ... Compared to 49 percent with general population programs*: Gold MS, Pomm R, Frost-Pineda K. "Urine testing confirmed, 5-year outcomes of impaired physicians." World Psychiatric Association; November 2004; Florence, Italy.

176 *But only 5.8 percent of doctors are Hispanic*: "Labor Force Statistics from the Current Population Survey." U.S. Bureau of Labor Statistics. https://www.bls.gov/cps/cpsaat11.htm | "Less than 3% of America's commercial pilots are Black. These men want to change that." *Philadelphia Tribune*. https://www.phillytrib.com/news/across_america/less-than-3-of-americas-commercial-pilots-are-black-these-men-want-to-change-that/article_74235f00-7265-529b-a066-1b7b714c9cbc.html

176 *implicit biases*: "Implicit Bias." National Institutes of Health. https://diversity.nih.gov/sociocultural-factors/implicit-bias | "Implicit Bias." Perception Institute. https://perception.org/research/implicit-bias/ | "Implicit Bias." Merriam Webster. https://www.merriam-webster.com/dictionary/implicit%20bias

176 *A 2005 study of hundreds of patients showed*: Chen I, Kurz J, Pasanen M, Faselis C, Panda M, Staton LJ, O'Rorke J, Menon M, Genao I, Wood J, Mechaber AJ, Rosenberg E, Carey T, Calleson D, Cykert S. "Racial differences in opioid use for chronic nonmalignant pain." *J Gen Intern Med* 2005 Jul;20(7):593–8. https://pubmed.ncbi.nlm.nih.gov/16050852/

176 *Another study similarly showed that physicians are twice as likely*: Staton LJ, Panda M, Chen I, Genao I, Kurz J, Pasanen M, Mechaber AJ, Menon M, O'Rorke J, Wood J, Rosenberg E, Faeslis C, Carey T, Calleson D, Cykert S. "When race matters: disagreement in pain perception between patients and their physicians in primary care." *J Natl Med Assoc* 2007 May;99(5):532–8. https://pubmed.ncbi.nlm.nih.gov/17534011/

177 *one of which was pain tolerance*: "Some medical students still think black patients feel less pain than whites." STAT News. https://www.statnews.com/2016/04/04/medical-students-beliefs-race-pain/ | "Black Americans are Systematically Under-Treated for Pain. Why?" University of Virginia Frank Batten School of Leadership and Public Policy. https://batten.virginia.edu/about/news/black-americans-are-systematically-under-treated-pain-why

179 *Race refers to inherited physical characteristics used to describe people*: "The Difference Between Race and Ethnicity." Verywell Mind. https://www.verywellmind.com/difference-between-race-and-ethnicity-5074205 | "What's the difference between race and ethnicity?" Live Science. https://www.livescience.com/difference-between-race-ethnicity.html

180 *Language is exactly that*: "Race, Ethnicity, and Language Data: Standardization for Health Care Quality Improvement." Agency for Healthcare Research and Quality (AHRQ). https://www.ahrq.gov/research/findings/final-reports/iomracereport/reldata4.html

180 *Sexuality or sexual orientation refers to*: "Sexual Orientation and Gender Identity Definitions." Human Rights Campaign (HRC). https://www.hrc.org/resources/sexual-orientation-and

NOTES

-gender-identity-terminology-and-definitions | "Sexual Orientation." Planned Parenthood. https://www.plannedparenthood.org/learn/sexual-orientation/sexual-orientation

180 *I've even seen other experts transform REaLS to REALD*: "Using REALD and SOGI to Identify and Address Health Inequities." Oregon Health Authority. https://www.oregon.gov/oha/EI/Pages/Demographics.aspx

182 *Everyday Discrimination Scale*: Williams DR, Yu Y, Jackson JS, Anderson NB. "Racial Differences in Physical and Mental Health: Socioeconomic Status, Stress, and Discrimination." *Journal of Health Psychology* 1997; 2(3):335–51 | "Everyday Discrimination Scale." David R. Williams, graduate school professor of public health at Harvard University. https://scholar.harvard.edu/davidrwilliams/node/32397

187 *Mindfulness app specifically for African Americans called Mindful You*: Watson-Singleton NN, Pennefather J, Trusty T. "Can a culturally responsive Mobile health (mHealth) application reduce African Americans' stress?: A pilot feasibility study." *Curr Psychol* 2023;42:1434–43. https://link.springer.com/article/10.1007/s12144-021-01534-9 | Black Fullness. https://www.blackfullness.com/

Chapter Six: Scrolling Toward Addiction

199 *Juul backstory*: "The Disturbing Focus of Juul's Early Marketing Campaigns." *Forbes*, November 16, 2018. https://www.forbes.com/sites/kathleenchaykowski/2018/11/16/the-disturbing-focus-of-juuls-early-marketing-campaigns/?sh=5fdbdb3514f9 | "4 Marketing Tactics e-cigarette companies use to target youth." Truth Initiative. https://truthinitiative.org/research-resources/tobacco-industry-marketing/4-marketing-tactics-e-cigarette-companies-use-target | "Silicon Valley's favorite e-cig company shut down its social media accounts—but Juul's advertising now has a life of its own." Insider Inc. https://www.businessinsider.com/why-juul-shut-down-social-media-facebook-instagram-vaping-2018-11 | "E-Cigarette Maker Juul Labs Is Shutting Down Its U.S. Facebook and Instagram Accounts." *Adweek*. November 13, 2018, https://www.adweek.com/performance-marketing/e-cigarette-maker-juul-labs-is-shutting-down-its-u-s-facebook-and-instagram-accounts/ | "Juul to pay nearly $440M to settle states' probe into marketing of vaping products for teens." *USA Today*, September 6, 2022. https://www.usatoday.com/story/news/health/2022/09/06/juul-settlement-marketing-teen-vaping/8003754001/

200 *In 2014, nearly 70 percent of middle and high school–aged children were exposed to*: "E cigarette Ads and Youth." Centers for Disease Control and Prevention (CDC). https://www.cdc.gov/vitalsigns/ecigarette-ads/index.html

200 *whiffs of smoke could taste like*: "Vape Juice & E-Liquids." Breazy. https://breazy.com/collections/juices

200 *By 2018, Juul, which held the vast majority of the e-cigarette market, was on track to become a billion-dollar company. They had increased their revenue 300 percent*: Fadus MC, Smith TT, Squeglia LM. "The rise of e-cigarettes, pod mod devices, and Juul among youth: Factors

NOTES

influencing use, health implications, and downstream effects." *Drug Alcohol Depend* 2019 Aug 1;201:85–93. https://www.ncbi.nlm.nih.gov/pmc/articles/PMC7183384/ | "Inside Juul Labs—how the vaping giant hooked its users and became a $15 billion company." CNBC. https://www.cnbc.com/2018/09/11/how-juul-became-a-15-billion-vaping-giant.html

200 *One study for eleven- to sixteen-year-old nonsmokers showed*: Vasiljevic M, Petrescu DC, Marteau TM. "Impact of advertisements promoting candy-like flavoured e-cigarettes on appeal of tobacco smoking among children: an experimental study." *Tob Control* 2016;25:e107–e112. https://tobaccocontrol.bmj.com/content/tobaccocontrol/25/e2/e107.full.pdf

201 *Their studies showed that exposure to social media posts*: Vogel EA, Ramo DE, Rubinstein ML, Delucchi KL, Darrow SM, Costello C, Prochaska JJ. "Effects of Social Media on Adolescents' Willingness and Intention to Use E-Cigarettes: An Experimental Investigation." *Nicotine Tob Res* 2021 Mar 19;23(4):694–701. https://pubmed.ncbi.nlm.nih.gov/31912147/ | Lee J, Tan AS, Porter L, Young-Wolff KC, Carter-Harris L, Salloum RG. "Association Between Social Media Use and Vaping Among Florida Adolescents, 2019." *Prev Chronic Dis* 2021;18:200550. https://www.cdc.gov/pcd/issues/2021/20_0550.htm

201 *One study showed that four out of five students overestimated*: Agaku IT, Odani S, Homa D, Armour B, Glover-Kudon R. "Discordance between perceived and actual tobacco product use prevalence among US youth: a comparative analysis of electronic and regular cigarettes." *Tob Control* 2019 Mar;28(2):212–9. https://pubmed.ncbi.nlm.nih.gov/29674512/

202 *Culture definition*: "What is culture?" *Live Science*. https://www.livescience.com/21478-what-is-culture-definition-of-culture.html | "Culture." *Encyclopedia Britannica*. https://www.britannica.com/topic/culture | "What Is Culture?" Boston University School of Public Health. https://sphweb.bumc.bu.edu/otlt/mph-modules/PH/CulturalAwareness/CulturalAwareness2.html

202 *Some research shows that country music songs have the highest reference to drug use*: "Drugs in Music—Analyzing Drug References in Musical Genres." Addictions.com. https://www.addictions.com/explore/drugs-in-music-analyzing-drug-references-in-musical-genres/

204 *But this was in the '70s when marijuana use*: "Blazing through the ages: Cannabis prevalent on campus in '70s." *The Pitt News*. https://pittnews.com/article/1116/arts-and-entertainment/blazing-through-the-ages-cannabis-prevalent-on-campus-in-70s/

207 *Young people who start using marijuana before the age of fourteen have increased risk*: "Teens." National Center for Injury Prevention and Control, Centers for Disease Control and Prevention (CDC). https://www.cdc.gov/marijuana/health-effects/teens.html

208 *CVS backstory*: "CVS President & CEO Larry Merlo speaks at The National Press Club." National Press Club Live. https://www.youtube.com/watch?v=FCC28RGzRwo | "How quitting tobacco reshaped CVS: Q&A with CEO Larry Merlo." *USA Today*, September 3, 2019. https://www.usatoday.com/story/money/2019/09/03/cvs-pharmacy-tobacco-sales-ceo

NOTES

-larry-merlo/2151148001/ | Polinski JM, Howell B, Gagnon MA, Kymes SM, Brennan TA, Shrank WH. "Impact of CVS Pharmacy's Discontinuance of Tobacco Sales on Cigarette Purchasing (2012–2014)." *Am J Public Health* 2017 Apr;107(4):556–62. doi: 10.2105/AJPH.2016.303612. Epub 2017 Feb 16. PMID: 28207340; PMCID: PMC5343689. | "When CVS stopped selling cigarettes, some customers quit smoking." Reuters, March 20, 2017. https://www.reuters.com/article/us-health-pharmacies-cigarettes/when-cvs-stopped-selling-cigarettes-some-customers-quit-smoking-idUSKBN16R2HY

208 *One of the largest threats to American public health in history*: "Tobacco." World Health Organization (WHO). https://www.who.int/news-room/fact-sheets/detail/tobacco

208 *Worldwide, tobacco kills 7 million people every single year and in the United States it takes the lives of nearly half a million annually*: "Diseases and Death." Office on Smoking and Health, National Center for Chronic Disease Prevention and Health Promotion (CDC). https://www.cdc.gov/tobacco/data_statistics/fact_sheets/fast_facts/diseases-and-death.html

208 *Consumer Value Stores, now known as CVS, has come a long way*: "CVS Health." *Supermarket News*. https://www.supermarketnews.com/companies/cvs-health

209 *Roughly 70 percent of the United States lives within three miles of a CVS*: "Creating Value by Transforming the Consumer Health Experience." CVS Health. https://s2.q4cdn.com/447711729/files/doc_events/2019/InvestorDay2019/2019-CVS-Investor-Day-Full-Presentation.pdf

209 *They would stop selling tobacco products in their stores because it was the right thing for a healthcare company to do*: "CVS stores to stop selling tobacco." CNN. https://www.cnn.com/2014/02/05/health/cvs-cigarettes/index.html

209 *rang the opening bell*: "CVS Health Rings the NYSE Opening Bell." YouTube. https://youtu.be/-mz3udN4GXw

209 *CVS Health's stock didn't tank. It actually rose. Steadily. For the next year*: "CVS Health Corp MarketSummary."Google.https://www.google.com/search?q=cvs+stock+over+past+ten+years

210 *Research found that 95 million fewer packs of cigarettes were sold across the country*: "When CVS stopped selling cigarettes, some customers quit smoking." Reuters. https://www.reuters.com/article/us-health-pharmacies-cigarettes/when-cvs-stopped-selling-cigarettes-some-customers-quit-smoking-idUSKBN16R2HY | "CVS President & CEO Larry Merlo speaks at The National Press Club." YouTube. https://www.youtube.com/live/FCC28RGzRwo

210 *The average smoker in markets where CVS had a significant presence purchased five fewer packs*: Polinski JM, Howell B, Gagnon MA, Kymes SM, Brennan TA, Shrank WH. "Impact of CVS Pharmacy's Discontinuance of Tobacco Sales on Cigarette Purchasing (2012–2014)." *American Journal of Public Health* 2017 Apr;107(4):556–62. https://www.ncbi.nlm.nih.gov

NOTES

/pmc/articles/PMC5343689/ | "Tobacco-free for five years." CVS Health. https://www.cvshealth.com/news/community/tobacco-free-for-five-years.html

210 *Prohibition backstory*: "Prohibition." History Channel, A&E Television Networks. https://www.history.com/topics/roaring-twenties/prohibition | Blocker JS Jr. "Did prohibition really work? Alcohol prohibition as a public health innovation." *American Journal of Public Health* 2006 Feb;96(2):233–43. https://www.ncbi.nlm.nih.gov/pmc/articles/PMC1470475/

210 *In 1995, California became the first state to ban smoking in every workplace and indoor public space*: "California Tobacco Laws that Reduce ETS Exposure." California Air Resources Board. https://ww2.arb.ca.gov/our-work/programs/environmental-tobacco-smoke/california-tobacco-laws-reduce-ets-exposure

211 *Studies have shown that the less Latinx immigrants who come to this country acculturate, the less risk they have for susceptibility to addiction*: Ojeda VD, Patterson TL, Strathdee SA. "The influence of perceived risk to health and immigration-related characteristics on substance use among Latino and other immigrants." *American Journal of Public Health* 2008 May;98(5): 862–8. https://www.ncbi.nlm.nih.gov/pmc/articles/PMC2374816/ | Flórez KR, Derose KP, Breslau J, Griffin BA, Haas AC, Kanouse DE, Stucky BD, Williams MV. "Acculturation and Drug Use Stigma Among Latinos and African Americans: An Examination of a Church-Based Sample." *J Immigr Minor Health* 2015 Dec;17(6):1607–14. https://www.ncbi.nlm.nih.gov/pmc/articles/PMC4512929/#R1

211 *Another study of more than 3,500 Asian Americans showed that US-born Asian Americans*: Lo CC, Cheng TC, Howell RJ. "The Role of Immigration Status in Heavy Drinking Among Asian Americans." *Substance Use & Misuse* 2014;49(8):932–40. https://www.tandfonline.com/doi/full/10.3109/10826084.2013.852578

213 *Created by the American Psychiatric Association (APA), the questionnaire is meant to help clinicians*: "Cultural Formulation Interview." American Psychiatric Association. https://www.psychiatry.org/File%20Library/Psychiatrists/Practice/DSM/APA_DSM5_Cultural-Formulation-Interview.pdf

220 *We've developed into beings who are overly influenced by those around us*: "Herd mentality: Are we programmed to make bad decisions?" University of Exeter. https://www.sciencedaily.com/releases/2014/12/141216212049.htm

220 *Herd mentality is neurobiologically hardwired into our brains*: Zhang W, Yang D, Jin J, Diao L, Ma Q. "The Neural Basis of Herding Decisions in Enterprise Clustering: An Event-Related Potential Study." *Front Neurosci* 2019;13:1175. https://www.frontiersin.org/articles/10.3389/fnins.2019.01175/full | Kameda T, et al. "The Concept of Herd Behaviour: Its Psychological and Neural Underpinnings." In Grundmann S, Möslein F, Riesenhuber K (eds.). *Contract Governance: Dimensions in Law and Interdisciplinary Research* (Oxford, 2015; online ed, Oxford Academic, 17 Sept. 2015). https://academic.oup.com/book/11486/chapter-abstract/160205905?redirectedFrom=fulltext

IMAGE CREDITS

220 *The same way that herds of animals move together knowing there is safety*: "Why do animals do what they do? Part 2: A herd is good." Michigan State University. https://www.canr.msu.edu/news/why_do_animals_do_what_they_do_part_2_a_herd_is_good | "Direct-Benefit Effect in Herd Behavior." Cornell University. https://blogs.cornell.edu/info2040/2012/10/29/direct-benefit-effect-in-herd-behavior/

220 *We mostly cluster together in urban areas rather than living isolated by ourselves*: "U.S. Cities Factsheet." Center for Sustainable Systems, University of Michigan, 2021, Pub. No. CSS09–06. https://css.umich.edu/publications/factsheets/built-environment/us-cities-factsheet | "68% of the world population projected to live in urban areas by 2050, says UN." United Nations Department of Economic and Social Affairs (UN DESA). https://www.un.org/development/desa/en/news/population/2018-revision-of-world-urbanization-prospects.html

227 *New Year's Eve, the Fourth of July, and Thanksgiving are the top three deadliest days of the year for drunk driving*: "2023's Most Dangerous Days for DUIs." MoneyGeek. https://www.moneygeek.com/insurance/auto/resources/most-dangerous-dui-days/

Image Credits

Cover art: Shutterstock.com: Melitas (profiles); Parrot Ivan (features)

Interior art: Getty Images: DigitalVision Vectors/bortonia: 3 (helix); iStock/Getty Images Plus: GetThis: 3 (body); grebeshkovmaxim: 3 (head); johnwoodcock: 238; speedmanstudio: 3 (gears); Shutterstock.com: melitas: 16, 126

Acknowledgments

People always ask me—how do you do it all? And my answer is always "I don't." My entire life, this book included, is made possible by a village that I am so deeply thankful for, I have tears in my eyes just thinking about it. In chronological order of appearance, thank you:

Mom—You are the quintessential mother and grandmother that I strive to emulate each day. I learned "human first" and compassion by watching you. I love you to the moon and back.

Dad—for being Founder and Commander of the Indianapolis Black Panther Militia and for raising us in our Kwanzaa community. I learned activism by watching you.

Modibo and Akosua—for being the most amazing siblings a girl could ask for. We were *Raised to Be Free*. Debo, we will keep fighting until you are.

Allison, Natalie, Keri, Janice, Cheryl, Renni, and Lisa—for being my best friends, safe place, and sense of belonging in high school, college, medical school, and beyond.

Trevor, David, Srishti, Bennett, Olivia, and the entire Oxeon Venture Studio and Town Hall Ventures teams—for asking the question: "Will the market invest in value-based OUD care?"

Corbin—for cofounding this amazing journey called Eleanor Health.

Our entire Eleanor team—for pouring your hearts and souls into our community members.

Andy Slavitt—for your unwavering support. And for introducing me to Jess and Steph at Lemonada Media who created In Recovery with Dr. Harrison (available wherever you get your podcasts, lol) and directly led to the opportunity to write this book.

ACKNOWLEDGMENTS

Jennifer Keene and the Octagon team—for being so passionate about people with addiction. For connecting me to the best collaborating author ever and for getting this book sold.

Lynya Floyd—for capturing my voice, my stories, my beliefs, my soapboxes, and my quirks. Your talent amazes me. Let's do it again, shall we?

Jessica Firger and the Union Square & Co. publishing team—for caring enough about people with addiction to publish this book. For supporting me and Lynya through the writing process. For super thoughtful edits. For creating a platform for this conversation.

Dr. Vincent J. Felitti, Dr. Christina Bethell, and Dr. Arline Geronimus, the researchers who provided not only moving stories and fascinating data, but also time for interviews to be a part of this book.

Every person whose story is in this book that I haven't mentioned—for being who you are, persisting and sharing your story.

Shirley—for loving me like a daughter without the in-law part. You are a gem.

Zahir and Nasir—for being a source of joy and pride too deep to describe. Being your mother will always be the most important thing I've done with my life. Love you!

Joel—for making me laugh, wiping my tears, sharing adventures, rubbing my head, listening to my rants, calling me on my BS, charging my car, holding down all the things while I travel, always saying yes to our next big opportunity, being the Dad to Zahir and Nasir that I always dreamt of, and for being my rock. I love you.

Index

A

abstinence, a104–106, 149–151, 203, 211, 213. *See also* Alcoholics Anonymous (AA)

ACE questionnaire. *See also* Adverse Childhood Experiences (ACE)
- on child sexual abuse, 68
- community-level stressors and, 74–77
- on depression and mental illnesses, 71
- on domestic abuse, 70
- evaluating responses to, 76–77
- expectations, 65–66
- on feeling nurtured, 69
- foster care, 76
- on household members in prison, 71
- Institutional Review Board rejecting, 59–60
- on meeting basic needs, 69
- on parents' separation/ divorce, 69–70
- on physical abuse, 68
- physical/emotional reactions to, 66
- problems with, 74–77
- stress levels, 66
- on substance use in home environment, 70–71
- on verbal abuse, 67–68

acquired risks
- biological, 5, 148–149, 152
- environmental, 5, 206, 208
- psychological, 5, 167, 172

Adderall, 142, 144–145

addict, persons with addiction vs, 12–13

addiction. *See also* preaddiction; severe addiction; substance use
- biological risks for, 132
- as chronic medical disease, 2
- as coded in DNA, 43–44, 50–51, 107
- as compulsive, 2
- defined, 1

identifying early warning signs of, 38–39
- metaphors, 116
- parts of the brain associated with, 28–32
- preventing (*See* addiction prevention)
- psychiatric evaluations for, 20–21
- recreational drug use leading to, 133
- reducing risks, 34
- risk of, 2–3, 54, 107–113, 123, 199–200
- from self-medicating, 133
- as treatable, 2
- treatment for, 20–21
- vulnerability to, 162
- website resources, 236–237

addiction family tree, 35, 238–239

addiction prevention
- behavioral awareness, 35–42
- conversations about (*See* conversation checklists)
- cutting use in half, 40–41
- family history awareness, 32–35
- getting support for yourself, 46–47
- reaching out for help, 39–40
- retaking CAGE questionnaire, 41
- talking to primary care physician, 41–42
- technology support, 42

ADHD, 142

adrenaline, natural, 142

Adverse Childhood Experiences (ACE). *See also* childhood trauma
- antidote to (*See* Positive Childhood Experiences (PCEs))
- data analysis, 60–61
- impact of abuse, by type, 59
- lack of diversity, 61–62
- limitations of, 61
- Philadelphia ACE Project, 75–76

questionnaire (*See* ACE questionnaire)
- science behind, 62–65
- strengths of, 61
- subsequent studies, 61–62

adversity, 167–168, 177. *See also* discrimination; weathering

Aetna, 207

African Americans. *See* people of color

alcohol, 146, 204

alcohol use disorder, 10–11, 120–122, 146

Alcoholics Anonymous (AA), 32, 81, 111, 189–190

Alexander, Bruce K., 94–97

allostatic load, 167

allyship, 221–222, 228–229

alprazolam, 136, 137, 139, 144

American Association for the Advancement of Science, 164

American Psychiatric Association (APA), 211–212

American Society of Addiction Medicine, 1, 100

amphetamines, 144–145

amygdala, 29–32, 75

Anda, Robert, 59

antianxiety medications. *See* benzodiazepines

anxiety. *See also* panic attacks
- easing, 124
- example of, 5, 216–217
- self-medicating for, 173
- treatment for, 132, 133–139, 153

apologies, 88

apps, 42

Archives of General Psychiatry, Valium advertisement in, 129–131

Asian Americans. *See* people of color

asthma, 4–5

Ativan, 136, 144

atomoxetine, 142

avoidance plans, 220–221, 224

INDEX

B

Bankhead neighborhood, Atlanta, 110
barbiturates, 135
behavioral awareness, 35–42
belonging, sense of, 81–82, 194–195
benzodiazepine withdrawal, 141
benzodiazepines, 133–139, 144, 145. *See also* opioids
Bethell, Christina, 78
biases, 175–176
binge drinkers, 20, 112, 214
biological risks, 34, 54, 62–65, 114–115, 205
Blackburn, Elizabeth, 167
blood pressure medications, 146
boundaries, 44, 46, 53, 225, 227, 228
brain function
    amygdala, 29–32, 75
    biological changes to, 151–152
    biological development of, 114
    dopamine pathway, 29–32, 69, 75, 103, 135, 145
    prefrontal cortex, 29–32, 75, 134, 145, 151
bupropion hydrochloride, 142

C

caffeine, 143
CAGE screening tool, 38–39, 41, 147–148, 156
California, 208
cannabis use disorder, 113
Carnegie Hill area, 109–112
Centers for Disease Control and Prevention, 22
Chicago, 110–111
childhood sexual assault, 58–59, 68
childhood trauma, 60–65, 72–74
Children's Defense Fund, 165
chronic illnesses, 4–5, 22–24, 133, 154–155
chronic stress, 168
cigarettes, 197–199, 204. *See also* tobacco; vaping
City Health Dashboard, 110
clonazepam, 136
cocaine, 7, 97, 143, 145
cocaine use disorder, 150, 155
codeine, 144
Community Catalyst, 100
community traditions, 81
community violence, 114

compassion
    for chronic illnesses, 23
    described, 7
    as first intervention, 224
    information combined with, 48–49
    setting boundaries, 44, 46
    transformational impact of, 27–28
compulsion to use, 13
Concerta, 144–145
concrete ceiling, 169–170
consequences, 13, 32, 44–45, 146, 172–177, 204
Consumer Value Stores. *See* CVS Health
conversation checklists
    for a child, 47–53
    differentiating addiction from the person, 49, 50
    for elementary school child, 49–51
    for family members/friends, 43–44
    for high school children, 52–53
    making connections, 49, 50–51
    for middle school children, 51
    nonjudgmental conversations, 45
    for a partner, 45–47
    for preschoolers, 48–49
coping mechanisms, 166, 170–172, 201
coping skills, 177, 215–216, 225
COVID pandemic, 98–99, 108–109, 139
Cultural Formulation Interview
    on barriers to getting help, 216–217
    on coping mechanisms, 215–216
    described, 211–212
    on identity, 212–213
    on other concerns, 215
    on practitioners and treatment already received, 216
    self-identifying substance use disorder risks, 214
    on support systems, 217–218
    on upbringing, 213
cultural revolution
    creating, 222, 231
    holiday festivities, 225–227

    teenage rites of passage, 222–225
    vacation getaways, 227–229
culturally relevant care, 211
culture
    of college, 202–203
    CVS Health and, 206–209
    government regulations influencing, 201–202, 208
    language use and, 200
    on a macro level, 199–200
    media influence on, 200–201
    on micro level, 200
    office/profession, 201
    overcoming influences of, 209–210
    as source of addiction risk, 199–200
    substance use temptations (*See* temptations)
    subversive impact of, 209–211
CVS Health, 206–209

D

daytime tranquilizers. *See* Valium
deep breathing, 31
deflecting, 90
delirium, 140–141
depression, 29, 42, 71, 78, 114, 156, 183
Desoxyn, 144–145
Dexedrine, 144–145
dexmethylphenidate, 144–145
dextroamphetamine, 144–145
Diagnostic and Statistical Manual of Mental Disorders: 5th Edition (DSM-V), 35–36
diazepam. *See* Valium
discrimination. *See also* biases; Everyday Discrimination Scale (EDS); microaggressions; racism
    ACE questions and, 74
    addiction risk tied to, 194
    example of, 5
    importance of PCEs, 168, 234
    negative consequences of, 182–183
    safe spaces shielding, 189, 194–195
    silence about, 186
    trauma of, 168–169, 172–173
DNA, 43–44, 50–51, 107, 114

INDEX

doctors. *See* physicians
domestic abuse, 70
dopamine deficiency, 105
dopamine pathway, 29–32, 69, 75, 103, 135, 145
drug overdoses, 135, 138, 140–141, 188, 204
drug rehab, 31
drug screenings, 223–224
drug use. *See* substance use
drug-drug interactions, 140–141

E
East Harlem, 109–112
Eleanor Health, 12, 37–38, 179–180, 234–235
electronic cigarettes, 197–199
emotions
  bypassing, 85
  censoring ourselves, 88
  deflecting, 90
  embracing silence, 91
  expressing, 85
  humor and, 90
  muting, 85
  physiological grounding techniques, 87
  recognizing, 86
  sharing with someone else, 87–89
  tears and, 91
  validating, 90
  when someone else is sharing, 89–91
enabling, 44, 45–46, 102
environment
  acquired environmental factors, 5, 206, 208
  addiction risk linked to, 123
  analyzing, 119–122
  biological changes, 114–115
  changing your, 120–122
  as a child, 121
  impact on substance use, 98, 120–121
  impacting DNA, 114
  learning from childhood, 116–118
  making intentional decisions about, 120
  power of, on health, 111
  safe, example of, 117
  vacations and, 118–119
environmental stress, 114
environmental triggers, 111–112
epigenetics, 114

ethnicity, 179
Everyday Discrimination Scale (EDS), 182–183, 184–185. *See also* discrimination
experimental psychology, 95
explicit biases, 175–176

F
Faces & Voices of Recovery (FAVOR), 100
false truths, 25–26
family history, awareness of, 32–35
family members
  chosen families, 80
  communicating with, 80
  conversation with, 43–44
  in prison, 71
  separation/divorce, 69–70
  sharing feelings with, 85
family tree, addiction, 35, 238–239
feelings. *See* emotions
Felitti, Vincent, 57–59
fentanyl, 144
Fentora, 144
fight-flight-freeze responses, 64, 133
Focalin, 144–145
food desert, 108–109
friendships. *See also* family members
  conversation with, 43–44
  finding, as an adult, 84
  as predictor of wellness, 82
  as support, 80–81
Frontiers in Behavioral Neuroscience, 97

G
GABA (chemical), 134
gambling game, 148–151
gender identity, 179–180
geography, impact on substance use, 112. *See also* culture
Geronimus, Arline T., 164–166. *See also* weathering
glass ceiling in the workplace, 169
"glass cliff", 169

H
health disparities by demographic groups, 175
healthcare professionals. *See* primary care physicians
heavy drinking, defined, 43

herd mentality, 218–219
heritability, 23–24, 54, 107, 205
Heritability of Chronic Illnesses chart, 22–23, 25
heroin, 47, 95–97, 103–104, 140, 216–217. *See also* opioids
heroin study, 95–97
high school, sense of belonging in, 81–82
holidays, 225–227
hotlines, 237
Houston, Whitney, 138
humor, 90
hydrocodone, 140, 144

I
Icahn School of Medicine, 149–150
implicit biases, 175–176
incest, 58
inherited risks, 6
Institutional Review Board, 59–60
insulin, 147
isolation living, 98–99

J
JAMA Pediatrics, 78
John Henryism, 181–182
Juul, 197, 198–199

K
Kaiser Permanente San Diego, 57
Klonopin, 136

L
language, 7–9, 15, 179, 200. *See also* words
Librium, 135
life expectancy, 110–111
Lil Wayne, 138
limbic system, 28–29
lorazepam, 136, 144
love languages, 82, 89

M
Magic Formula™ for recovery, 3, 32–33, 39–42, 106, 234
mantras, 32
marginalized communities, 169, 174–175, 189. *See also* people of color
marijuana use, 11, 202–205
McEwen, Bruce, 167
medical cannabis dispensaries, 113

INDEX

medical professionals. *See* physicians
medications, fear/suspiciousness of, 143–146
meditation, 63
mental health, reducing risk of, 79
mentors, 83
Merlo, Larry J., 206
Metadate, 144–145
methamphetamine, 144–145
Methylin, 144–145
methylphenidate, 144–145
methylphenidate hydrochloride, 144–145
microaggressions, 170–171, 180–182, 189. *See also* discrimination; racism
Mindful You (app), 176–177
mindfulness app, 176–177, 186–187
mindfulness meditation practice, 31
Monroe, Marilyn, 135
morphine study, 94–97
morphine sulfate, 144
Moving to Opportunity study, 114–115
MS Contin, 144

N

narcotics. *See* opioids
Narcotics Anonymous, 81, 189–190
National Institute on Alcohol Abuse and Alcoholism, 43
National Institute on Drug Abuse (NIDA) study, 97
National Survey of Children's Health survey, 78
natural adrenaline, 142
Nembutal, 135
neuroplasticity, 63
New York City, 109–110
nicotine, 34
North American Association for the Study of Obesity conference, 57–58
nurturing, 69, 75, 219

O

obesity, childhood trauma and, 57–59
open-ended questions, 191
opioid crisis, 232–233

opioids, 139–142, 144. *See also* benzodiazepines
ORT (Opioid Risk Tool), 147–148, 149, 156
overdoses. *See* drug overdoses
oxazepam, 144
oxycodone hydrochloride, 144
OxyContin, 144

P

pain clinics, 139–140
pain tolerance, 175–176
painkillers. *See* opioids
panic attacks, 137, 172–173. *See also* anxiety
partners, 45–47, 83
patterns, 40, 64
PCEs. *See* Positive Childhood Experiences (PCEs)
peer pressure, 51, 217–218, 220–221
People, Places, and Things mantra, 111
people of color, 61–62, 108–109, 165–168, 173–177, 186–187, 190
people-first language, 12
perceptions, 181
Percocet, 140, 144
perseverance, 115–116
personal space, 192
persons with addiction, addict vs, 12–13
Philadelphia ACE Project, 75–76
physical abuse, 68
physicians, 41–42
 biases of, 10, 175–176
 building a partnership with, 156–157
 communicating with, 41–42
 pressure to prescribe medications, 158
 recovery programs for, 175
 substance use disorder risk and, 154–156
 talking to, 152–154
 underestimating Black patients' pain, 175–176
 Valium risk, discussion on, 132
physiological grounding techniques, 87
physiological stressors, 168–169
Planned Parenthood, 165
Positive Childhood Experiences (PCEs)
 in adulthood, 79
 belonging, sense of, 81–82
 chosen families, 80
 described, 77–78
 questionnaire, 79–83
 reducing mental health risks, 79
 support systems, 80
potheads, 11
preaddiction, 36–42, 54–55, 124. *See also* addiction
prefrontal cortex, 29–32, 75, 134, 145, 151
prescription medications, 132–133, 157–161
prescription medications list, 155–156
present, being, 191
primary care physicians. *See* physicians
privacy protections, 153
prohibition, 208
psychiatric evaluations, 20–21
psychological stress, 114
psychological trauma, 63–64
PTSD (post-traumatic stress disorder), 106, 202

R

racism, 168–172, 175–176. *See also* discrimination; microaggressions
Rat Park experiment, 95–99. *See also* substance use myths
Reagan, Nancy, 94
REaLS framework, 178–179
rebound anxiety, 134–135
recovery, 100–101, 104–105, 148–151
recreational drug use, 104, 123–124, 204
REGaLS framework, 179–181, 187–188, 212–213
rehabilitation centers, 121
relapses, 13–15, 24–25, 111–112, 151, 175, 229
religious beliefs, 217
resources, 236–237
Restoril, 136
re-traumatization, 187, 188, 192
risk mitigation plan, 158–159
Ritalin, 142, 144–145
Roche (pharmaceutical company), 131
"rock bottom", 101–102

INDEX

S

safe spaces, 189–193
"safe word", 52
safety, sense of, 83
self-medicating, 133, 143–146, 202–203
Serax, 144
severe addiction, 36–37. *See also* addiction
sexual assault, 58–59, 72–74
sexuality/sexual orientation, 179
silence, embracing, 91
Simon Fraser University, 94
Skinner box, 95–96, 98, 100, 105, 118–119, 121
sleep disorders, 133
social drinkers, 20
St. Kitts, 19–20
Stellar, Eliot, 167
stimulants, 64, 142–143, 144–145
Strattera, 142
stress, 5, 66–67, 99, 114, 168–169. *See also* chronic stress
substance abuse, 9–12, 38–39
substance use. *See also* addiction
  apps for, 236
  artists and, 201
  behavioral response from, 64
  benefits of, 105–107, 124
  biological changes from, 160
  controlled, 104–105
  as coping mechanism, 170–172
  in home environment, 70–71
  muting emotions with, 85
  myths about (*See* substance use myths)
  as normal behavior, 11, 105
  physical environment's impact on, 98
  recovery factors, 100–101
  recreational, 104, 123–124
  substance abuse vs., 10–11
  temptations (*See* temptations)
  use patterns, 40
substance use disorders
  access to care, 174–175
  categories of, 35–36
  diagnosis criteria, 36
  in marginalized communities, 174–175
  of people of color, 173–174
  prescription pills increasing, 132–133
  recovery factors, 100–101, 104–105
  risks of, 154–156
Substance Use Journal, 40, 240
substance use myths
  automatic addiction to drugs, 103–105
  drug use is abnormal, 105–107
  hitting "rock bottom" for behavior change, 101–102
  people don't care about themselves, 99–101
Sullenberger, Sully, 29
support systems, 80, 121, 167, 183, 217–218, 233

T

tears, 91
technology support for addiction prevention, 42
teen pregnancy, 164–166
teenage rites of passage, 222–225
teetotalers, 20
telehealth, 178–179, 186
telomeres, 167
temazepam, 136
temptations
  addiction risk linked to, 230
  in culture, 230
  holidays, 225–227
  teenage rites of passage, 222–225
  vacation getaways, 227–229
therapeutic benefits of drugs, 147
tobacco, 206
translational research, 98
trauma-informed care, 180, 187. *See also* re-traumatization
triggers, 5
twelve-step programs. *See* Alcoholics Anonymous (AA)

U

United States Census Bureau, 110
United States Small-Area Life Expectancy Project (USALEEP), 110
University of Michigan, 164
unsafe space, 83
U.S. Department of Health and Human Services, 78

V

vacation getaways, 227–229
validation, 90
Valium, 129–134, 144
vaping, 197–199
verbal abuse, 67–68
vervet monkey population, 19–20, 21–22
Vicodin, 140, 144
visualization exercises, 32

W

warning signs of addiction, 9, 35, 38–39, 43, 47
Watson-Singleton, Natalie N., 186
weathering, 166–167, 194
websites, resource, 236–237
Wellbutrin, 142
Western medicine, 59
white-collar aspirin. *See* Valium
Williams, David R., 182
Williamson, David, 59
withdrawal, 135, 138, 141, 146–147
words, psychological power of, 8–9

X

Xanax, 136, 137, 139, 144

Z

Zanzibars, 138
zip codes, 107–113
ZNA, 107–113

About the Author

Dr. Nzinga Harrison is the Chief Medical Officer and Cofounder of Eleanor Health, an innovative company that provides compassionate care, a whole-person approach, and evidence-based treatment for individuals experiencing substance use disorders. A double board–certified physician in addiction medicine and psychiatry, her background includes a BS from Howard University, an MD from the University of Pennsylvania, and residency training at Emory University. Dr. Harrison holds adjunct faculty appointments at the Morehouse School of Medicine Department of Psychiatry and is cofounder of Physicians for Criminal Justice Reform, Inc.

As an internationally recognized, award-winning educator and advocate for mental health and addiction, Dr. Harrison has appeared for speaking engagements at the request of prestigious organizations and institutions including the American Society of Addiction Medicine, the American Psychiatric Association, the National Council for Mental Wellbeing, Black Psychiatrists of America, and Harvard Business School. Her expertise has been showcased in the media for outlets such as *NPR*, *BBC London Newsday Radio*, *Focus Atlanta TV*, and more. Online and print articles about Dr. Harrison have reached international audiences in publications like the *Huffington Post*, *The Hill*, and *She Knows*. She is also the featured expert in the award-winning feature documentary film on addiction, *Tipping the Pain Scale*. A married mother of two, she currently lives outside of Atlanta, Georgia.